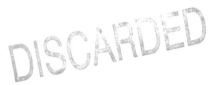

Praise for Sarah Reynold's professional organising work

'Sarah is brilliant! Her work goes beyond organising your physical space, and it declutters and clears your mind to discern what is really important to you. The benefits and rewards of the process ripple through every aspect of your life.'

SEAN WALL, KILDARE

'Sarah came into my home to help me declutter, purge and prepare for a move to a new country – but what she did was much more than that. Her work helped me understand how my mind functioned and how I lived along with my family so we could create spaces that felt both organised and functional whilst also feeling cosy and lived in. Our family now has a more calm and organised home.'

LESLIE ST LAWRENCE, SWITZERLAND

'With Sarah's amazing assistance we were able to do a complete and long overdue declutter of my five-bedroomed house. Her suggestions, advice and storage solutions were fantastic and now everything has a home.'

ANNE MARIE SUDWAY, DUBLIN

'Sarah has organising down to a science but she is also sensitive and caring in her approach to the work. Thanks to Sarah I now have systems which work to make sure my house stays organised.'

AISLING DAVENPORT, DUBLIN

About the Author

Sarah Reynolds is an organising expert and the owner of Organised Chaos.

Prior to establishing her business, Sarah worked in television for over ten years across many genres from entertainment to drama.

During a leave of absence, she undertook training in New York with Julie Morgenstern, America's number-one professional Organiser and regular contributor to the Oprah show, before returning home to set up her dream business.

Sarah helps home owners and businesses reach their full potential through effective organisation. Through her passion and practical solutions, her clients move from feeling overwhelmed to calm and in control. She transforms oppressive spaces into functional, productive and stylish places to live and work.

Sarah has shared her expertise on organisation and productivity worldwide through Irish, Canadian and US media. She is a regular speaker at nationwide events on the topic of home and workplace organisation.

Sarah studies singing in her spare time and loves everything to do with musical theatre.

She lives in Dublin, Ireland.

Find out more about Sarah and keep up to date with what's she's doing here:

www.organisedchaos.ie

Instagram.com/organisedchaosireland

Facebook.com/organisedchaosireland

Organised

Simple ways to declutter your house,
your schedule and your mind

SARAH REYNOLDS

GILL BOOKS

Gill Books
Hume Avenue
Park West
Dublin 12

www.gillbooks.ie

Gill Books is an imprint of M.H. Gill and Co.

© Sarah Reynolds 2017

978 07171 7556 7
All images © iStock and the author,
except page p. 85, © Polka Dot / Getty Images Plus
Edited by Jane Rogers
Printed by L&C Printing Group, Poland

This book is typeset in 11.5 on 14pt Bembo Regular.

5 4 3 2 1

To my parents, Eithne and
Dermot, for their constant love,
support and wisdom.

And for always encouraging me
to write.

Contents

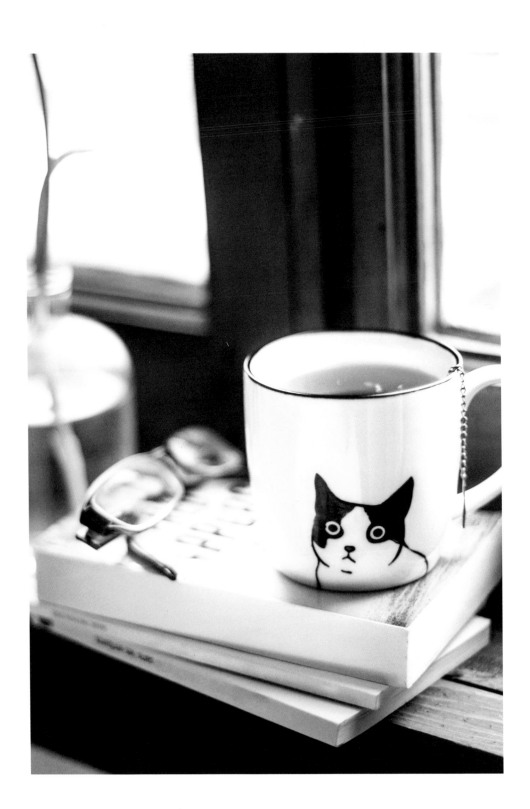

INTRODUCTION

·

'CHANGE IS HARD AT FIRST,
MESSY IN THE MIDDLE AND
GORGEOUS AT THE END.'

ROBIN SHARMA

·

I have two photos of me at home. One is a 'before' shot of my bedroom and the other is the tidy 'after' shot. I was eleven years old when those photos were taken. I'm often asked, 'Have you always been organised?' and the simple answer is 'Yes'. But when is life ever that simple? When I was fifteen, I was watching *Oprah* with my mother when Julie Morgenstern came on to discuss professional organising, her book and her business. Here was someone building a business doing what I loved doing. I was so inspired.

While I kept that interview and the idea of a business in the back of my mind, school had to be finished first, followed by university, which lead me down the path of getting a 'proper job', first in human resources and then in television where I stayed for ten years. At the age of thirty I decided to take a year's leave of absence and finally got to attend a training course with Julie in New York. I came back to Ireland, built a website and Organised Chaos was born. At thirty-four, having spent the previous three years double-jobbing, working on the business evenings and weekends, I decided to take the leap and go full time with the business. I left a permanent and pensionable job. I left friends I loved working with and financial security. My job had been like a second home to me. I knew the place inside out. I left it all for a future I thought I could see, but the reality turned out very different.

At thirty-five, my engagement and relationship of six years ended. With a new business and a broken heart, life didn't feel very organised any more. I was stressed, overwhelmed, sad and lonely, but I had to keep going. I had to make ends meet. My life had become organised chaos. My life was changing at a time and age that really wasn't ideal, and this most certainly wasn't part of the plan.

When people call me to organise their home or workplace, they think they're about to declutter and organise all the possessions they own. What they don't realise is that they're about to learn so much more about themselves. The essence of what I do is to help people through change. Change messes up our space, our schedules and ourselves. I was experiencing that myself. I recognised that I was going through this change and it was time for me to get back to basics, take back control, take care of myself and find space for some enjoyment. Get organised, essentially.

As writer and leadership speaker Robin Sharma says, 'Change is hard at first, messy in the middle and gorgeous at the end'. This isn't only true of change; it happens every time you get organised. It's really hard to get started. It gets worse before it gets better. And then it's gorgeous at the end.

Organised Chaos helps you to organise your outer environment at home or at work, so that you gain inner calm and control. As you will see through these pages, getting organised for me has always been about comfort. It's not about perfection, minimalism, or aiming to make your home look as if it jumped from the pages of a glossy magazine. It's about making your space work for you, not against you. It's organising for a reason – to achieve something; not doing it because you feel you have to.

The book is divided into four parts. It starts with yourself – because doesn't everything? In this part I explain why and how disorganisation and clutter build up and what role our habits and decisions play in this. Then we look at some goals that will keep us on track throughout the book and as you organise your space.

Part II is about your schedule because you'll never organise anything if you don't make time for it. A lot of disorganisation in our space comes from our time management anyway, so we address that here.

Once you've found time in your hectic life, we can get stuck in and clear space. Part III covers the main rooms I am called to help with in people's homes and how to declutter and organise them.

Finally, in Part IV, we come full circle and return to ourselves. We check in again with our habits and our commitment to the process so that the organisation is maintained over the long term.

Like any lifestyle change, getting started can seem overwhelming, and the process needs commitment to see it through. It's not easy, but you're up for a challenge, right? Sometimes we just have to take a deep breath, let go of whatever is holding us back and hope for the best. So let's get started. You're about to feel so much better.

Thank you for reading the book and I hope you enjoy it.

Happy organising!

Sarah

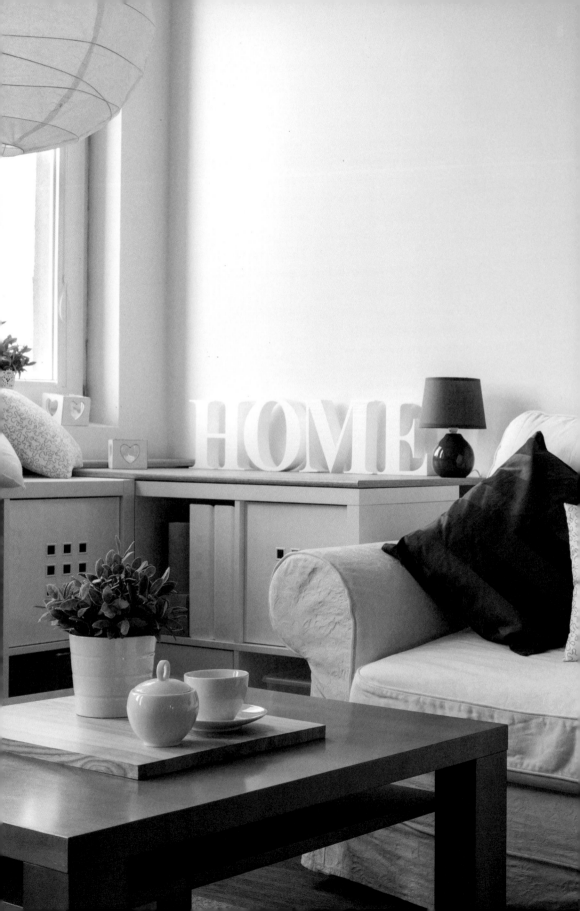

Part I

Yourself

.

'REMEMBER,
THE ONLY CONSTANT IN LIFE
IS CHANGE.'

BUDDHA

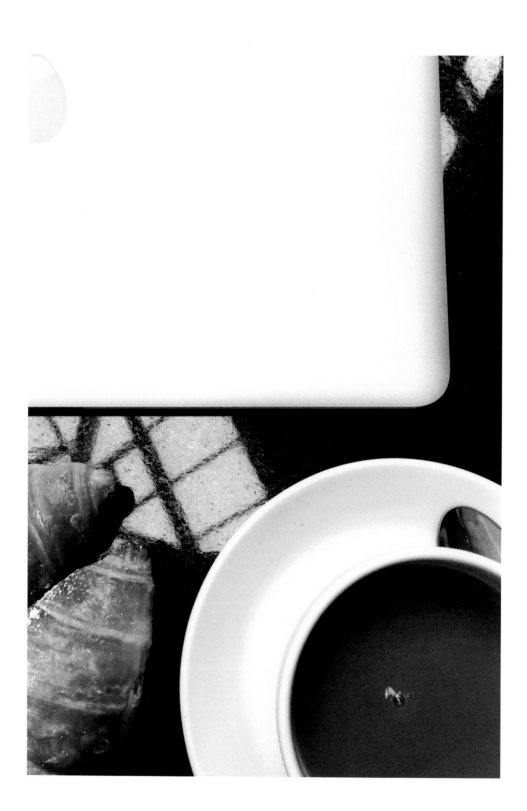

I

HABITS

·

**EVERY DAY JANE WALKS IN THROUGH
THE FRONT DOOR, DUMPS THE POST
FROM THE FLOOR ONTO THE CONSOLE,
AND THROWS HER COAT OVER
THE BANISTERS.**

·

Eric, her husband, and the kids arrive later that
evening and everything ends up on the hall floor
or the console. The mess drives Jane crazy.

·

If someone is missing their wallet, it might be in a coat pocket hanging on the banisters. More often than not, those things aren't in fact in the hall and the stress and time it takes to find them causes arguments and upset. The hall needs some organisation but there just isn't time.

Amy walks through the front door, dumps the post in the letter tray and hangs the coat under the stairs. John, her husband, and the kids arrive in later that evening. John throws his keys on a tray on the console and the kids put their bags under the stairs. John needs to pay the TV licence and finds it in the letter tray. The kids need their shin guards for rugby tomorrow and collect them from the basket of sports gear in the hall console. The hall is organised so that the way it's used goes unnoticed. There's nothing special about it, which is what makes it special.

Both scenarios are about family habits. In both scenarios, people have habits around how they use their stuff and their things. Neither is necessarily right or wrong. Unless one is causing stress and upset. That's when habits are no longer good habits.

If we want to make any lifestyle change, we first need to examine our current behaviour and habits. Achieving anything – getting fit, building a business, organising a house – requires setting up good habits. We know that simply wanting something to happen won't make it happen. A new habit, combined with a strong mindset, becomes fixed in our daily life and grows. However, sticking to a new habit isn't necessarily easy.

In his book *The Power of Habit*, Charles Duhigg explains the habit loop. Our brain registers a cue in our environment, and we then follow a certain routine in order to achieve a certain reward. Cues can be either positive or negative. He uses our phones and exercise as examples.

With our phones, as soon as the notification pings, our brain wants us to respond. This need builds up until we look at our phone. Our brain is rewarded with the satisfaction of knowing what was in the message. But doing this on demand, instead of at a time that suits us, results in a negative outcome: lack of focus, distraction from more important things, lower productivity.

If we exercise enough, we start to crave the endorphins, or the sense of achievement, and that's enough to make exercise a habit. This has positive results: good health, energy, motivation. The craving for the reward creates the habit (Duhigg, pp. 50-51).

I wanted to learn more about our organised mind, so I sat down with Dr Michael Keane of Actualise Clinic, based in Dublin City University. Actualise specialises in neurofeedback training, a scientifically validated method of 'brain training' that helps the brain to learn how to work in a more efficient way.

Michael Keane is a neuroscientist, psychologist and business owner and he recently finished his first year of graduate medicine (and you thought you were busy!). He says, 'everything is about organisation. There's no other way. My life as it stands is very well scheduled.' Given that he has two full-time jobs and an expanding practice, I wasn't surprised.

We discussed the idea of intermittent reinforcement in relation to our behaviour. He explained that the classic case in psychology is gambling. Every week we buy a lottery ticket and every week we don't win. The same is true of slot machines. We keep feeding money into them because each time we do there's a chance that we might win. Every now and then we win a small amount and that's enough of a reward to keep going. We are positively reinforced to keep up the habit.

So how does this psychology work in relation to our clutter? You might relate to the following scenarios.

It's the end of the day and you're getting ready for bed. Night after night, your clothes end up on the chair in the corner of the bedroom. Again and again you tell yourself, 'I have to clear that up' or, 'I need to get rid of that chair' or, 'This room is a mess. I'll never get around to sorting it out.' Looking at this mountain of clothes is irritating, almost upsetting, and the thought of clearing it is daunting. But you're trapped in your habit.

The cue each evening is the bed, the book, the need for sleep. Your routine is to get into bed as quickly as possible. The reward is rest. You crave rest, so this trumps putting the clothes away. Or perhaps you hate tidying, so you are getting satisfaction that the chair allows you to put off what you hate doing for another night.

You are positively reinforced because the chair will hold the mess for another night. Because, while it's not ideal, you will be able to find an outfit on the chair tomorrow morning. Because putting the clothes on the chair means that you don't have to open the wardrobe, so you are not reminded of the clutter in there. All of that plus a warm, cosy bed and a night's sleep ahead is enough of a reward to keep up the behaviour.

Now imagine early morning at home. Everyone always runs late. There are fights over what to eat for breakfast, you can't get the eldest out of bed and someone is always looking for something, from gym gear to their calculator. It's mayhem every morning. Because you leave late you always run into morning traffic, which adds stress to the journey. And yet, bar the odd morning, everyone arrives just about on time. You hate the stress and arguments that dominate the start of your day, but nothing changes.

There is always a pay-off. You are gaining something from not tidying and organising. It is only when the stress that clutter creates exceeds the stress of sorting it out that you will do something about it.

Behaviour that is least likely to change is behaviour that gets reinforced every now and then. Michael Keane says, 'The reward you get from intermittent reinforcement never goes away. People only stop [their behaviour] when it's very clear that there will be no benefit. If you were punished for the behaviour, it would extinguish the behaviour. But too often you get away with it.' But is the constant stress not the punishment? He explains, 'The relief only comes because the stress is there. The stress is punitive, but there is enough relief in those intermittent times to make the reward worth the stress. There isn't enough punishment from the stress because the stress is relieved straight away.' So until you get to a point where the punishment is greater than the relief, the behaviour remains.

Anthony Robbins, in his book *Awaken the Giant Within*, reiterates this psychology: 'one of the things that turns virtually anyone around is reaching a pain threshold. This means experiencing pain at such an intense level that you know you must change now – a point at which your brain says, "I've had it, I can't spend another day, not another moment, living or feeling this way"' (Robbins, p. 125).

For an organised person, seeing a clear desk, or arriving on time, is the reinforcement they need. That calmer state when they get to an appointment on time, or the enjoyment of working in a tidy office, gives enough reinforcement to continue the behaviour of organising and tidying. The physical environment makes them happy, so they keep doing the act (of organising) in order to keep them feeling happy.

An organised person may feel that they have enough to be worried about already; they don't want to be worried about losing their keys or having to wade through dozens of digital files to find the one they want. The control and calmness that a tidy external environment or a manageable schedule gives an organised person pushes them to create solutions.

For the majority of people, however, while they may feel disorganised, they probably don't feel disorganised enough to make any change.

That is, of course, until something happens. A major life event that throws everything into chaos.

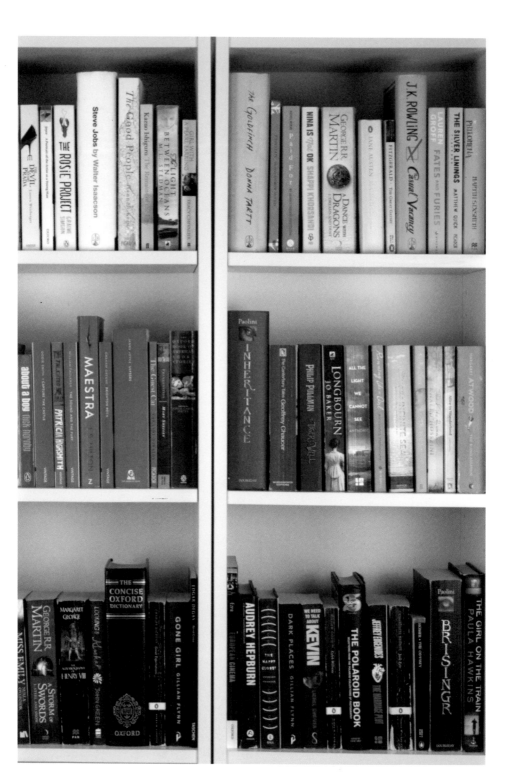

2

LIFE TRANSITIONS

·

LIFE CAN TAKE A TURN AT A MOMENT'S NOTICE.

·

Our family members or friends can get sick, injured, even die, and we're thrown into a tailspin. We can lose our jobs, get divorced, watch our kids emigrate; all big stressors in our lives. These situations challenge our ability to cope, bring anxiety into our lives and make us feel overwhelmed. Every one of my clients has come to me as a result of a transition in their lives.

·

I am contacted because the kitchen is full or there are toys everywhere or they're overwhelmed by their attic space. But the reason why these issues have arisen is because of a period of transition they have gone through recently or are about to go through.

CHANGE

Life changes affect the organisation of our home and highlight our own ability to organise ourselves. Our routines are thrown into disarray as we try to keep up with a new set of circumstances – sometimes sudden and not of our doing.

Life events that lead to a period of transition include:

- ILLNESS/HEALTH ISSUES – EITHER THE PERSON THEMSELVES OR A MEMBER OF THEIR FAMILY
- MOVING HOUSE
- RENOVATING THE HOME
- MARRIAGE
- BIRTH OF CHILDREN
- A CHILD/CHILDREN WITH A DISABILITY
- AGEING PARENTS
- CHILDREN LEAVING HOME
- RETIREMENT
- LOSING A JOB
- CHANGING JOB
- STARTING OR CLOSING A BUSINESS
- SEPARATION/DIVORCE
- END OF A RELATIONSHIP
- DEATH OF PARENTS
- DEATH OF SIGNIFICANT OTHER, FAMILY MEMBER OR FRIEND

What if before the bad news or new challenge, you were already losing your keys, forgetting to pay bills, missing appointments and fighting with your wardrobe? Disorganisation in your time and space was already a factor in your life; now it's exacerbated because of this mountain that has risen up along your path.

Incorporating organisation into your life – your time, home and work spaces – gets rid of all those nasty irritations that build up and build up. When you are faced with a challenge, whether it's a bad day at work, a car accident or something worse, your brain has more ability and space to deal with it if it isn't taken up with dealing with all the other smaller stressors that disorganisation brings.

Life's troubles are going to test your organisation anyway. When you're sad, angry or afraid, you will forget your keys, a bill, an appointment. But *having systems of organisation already in place can help*. Forgetting your keys will be a once-off. You'll remember to pay the bills promptly. Fixing those smaller stresses will be minor and allow you to focus your time and energy on the bigger issues.

If a life change is big enough, it usually involves a significant period of time – sometimes years – of decision-making, fighting to be heard, trying to cope and dealing with different people. We get worn out. When we come out at the other end, our battle wounds mean that we want to avoid making mistakes with any decisions from now on. That usually results in us not doing anything. Things stagnate. If things stagnate and decisions stall for long enough, clutter builds up. If we are still in the thick of this life change, feeling overwhelmed by everything can lead to paralysis. Nothing really gets done; life doesn't seem to move on one way or the other.

A disorganised home or office can result in feelings of being overwhelmed, anxiety, frustration and resentment. Frustrated by the mess and lack of space, we don't enjoy our home any more. This property that we worked so hard to get and to hold on to doesn't make us happy.

We leave it at every given opportunity. We'd rather eat out every night than face the kitchen. We fight with our partner over the mess, or get irritated with the kids, who won't tidy up. We work all week and resent having to spend the weekend cleaning the house. We never have enough time with those we love, rarely see our friends, can't find time for exercise and we don't remember the last time we did something for ourselves. Our money is going on eating out, cleaners and late payment fees. There's a constant feeling of catching up but never getting anywhere. Feelings of extreme tiredness, self-doubt, self-criticism and being overwhelmed lead to mounting levels of stress. If we're lucky we only have back pain, headaches and allergies to contend with.

Organisation — or lack of it — highlights change. Sometimes we have an active part in this change; sometimes the rug is pulled from under us. We are forced to re-prioritise and reflect. We realise we have limited time, limited resources, limited energy, limited help.

HOW BECOMING ORGANISED HELPS

Changes in your life may highlight areas in your physical environment that aren't working and aspects of your wellbeing that are suffering. You are getting further and further away from what makes you feel comfortable, and you want to restore some level of equilibrium. Getting organised is about comfort. It's not about having everything lined up in perfect order and alphabetised. If you have the time, energy and patience you can bring your organisation up to those levels, but for the average person's day-to-day life, organisation can be achieved with a lot less effort.

When a client contacts me, I begin with an initial consultation. Every consultation has resulted in the client changing how they perceived their environment. Suddenly, they are more aware of their space, what they are doing with their possessions, what is irritating them and why. They gain greater awareness of how they interact with their environment and how that interaction affects the way that environment is organised. Then they're motivated to examine their current behaviour around getting organised, and they haven't even lifted a finger yet.

In *The Power of Habit*, Charles Duhigg discusses how seemingly simple changes can affect us, suggesting that 'making your bed every morning is correlated with better productivity, a greater sense of wellbeing and stronger skills at sticking with a budget. It's not that a family meal or a tidy bed causes better grades or less frivolous spending. But somehow those *initial shifts start chain reactions that help other good habits* take hold' (Duhigg 2013, p.109).

If I'm coming in to help a client sort out their wardrobe following a divorce or the death of a partner, the temptation is to think that we are only dealing with the clothes themselves. But what I'm actually doing is helping the client adjust to their new life as a single person, saying goodbye to a certain way of life. As we go through the clothes, any resistance they feel is not because of the garment itself, but because they're having to let go and are getting closer to the other side of this transition. That can be very difficult, depending on what stage of grief they are at.

The same can be said for baby clothes. The difficulty is not the baby clothes in themselves; it's the 'what ifs', the regrets, wishing it was different. Some life transitions are positive – a new job, the arrival of a baby, moving into your dream house. These scenarios also shine a light on our surroundings, and sometimes we don't like what we see. We already have a lot of stress with a new baby, or organising a renovation or house move, so we don't want the additional stress of disorganisation and clutter.

Dr Keane mentions new parents and how they often become the most organised they have ever been. This is because, alongside this new life, everything else pales into insignificance. In the work environment, for example, a new parent will make a change to their organisation when they realise they've just spent 10 minutes looking for a file when they could have had an extra 10 minutes with their new baby.

When you think about it, *anything to do with our wellbeing starts with getting organised.*

To lose weight, we need to look at our food intake. But what exactly does that mean? It means finding the time to write a shopping list so that we don't buy the same unhealthy food we're used to. It's knowing where the pen and paper are to write the list in the first place. It's finding time to get to the supermarket to buy the food instead of calling for a takeaway. It's finding time to prepare meals and locating the Tupperware without having to empty every kitchen cupboard.

If we're concerned about our mental health, we need to get ourselves organised to make that initial phone call to a counsellor. Making appointments and finding the time for them is also part of the deal.

Even taking up a hobby or enjoying more time with family starts with organising our daily life. We have to organise our finances to pay for the art class. We have to organise cleaning the house so that we don't have to do it at the weekend and can go to the zoo instead.

If we can manage our time and organise our lives today a little bit better than we did yesterday, it makes us feel more in control. It allows us to factor in activities and tasks that we enjoy, are good for us, or that we need to do but had been putting off.

WHEN YOU THINK ABOUT IT, ANYTHING TO DO WITH OUR WELLBEING STARTS WITH GETTING ORGANISED.

I want to introduce you to the benefits of decluttering and the enjoyment that organisation can bring. I've worked with clients suffering from exhaustion, back pain, asthma and many other health issues. They are surrounded by so much stuff that just looking at it causes a lot of anxiety. Living in a home where you can't find anything, where every surface has something on it, where drawers are broken and the contents of cupboards fall out on top of you, where everyone is chasing their tails and there are constant arguments around possessions, cannot be good for your health.

Organisation is not going to take all your problems away. It's not going to make a child better, or ease the stress of minding an elderly parent, or make you feel less lonely when your heart is breaking. What it will do, though, is give you some breathing space; a little order in a world where you feel there is none. It reduces the amount of cleaning you have to do; it saves you money; it means that you don't have to nag so much; it enables you to find what you need when you need it; it means that you know where you're going and when, and what you're doing. There's just space. *Physical, emotional, mental space.*

Incorporating some organisation into your lifestyle will help return you to a state of comfort. The level of organisation you need or wish to achieve depends on your goals and your time. It's all in your hands.

Decluttering is the necessary evil you have to go through in order to create space. After that there is the art of organisation. This is the fun part if you can stick with the process. This is the part where you get to design new systems and new ways to use your time and space, create new habits, adopt a new lifestyle. It's the part where you can go shopping again (wisely!).

Stick with it long enough and it'll truly get under your skin; it will simply become something you do, and then you'll love it.

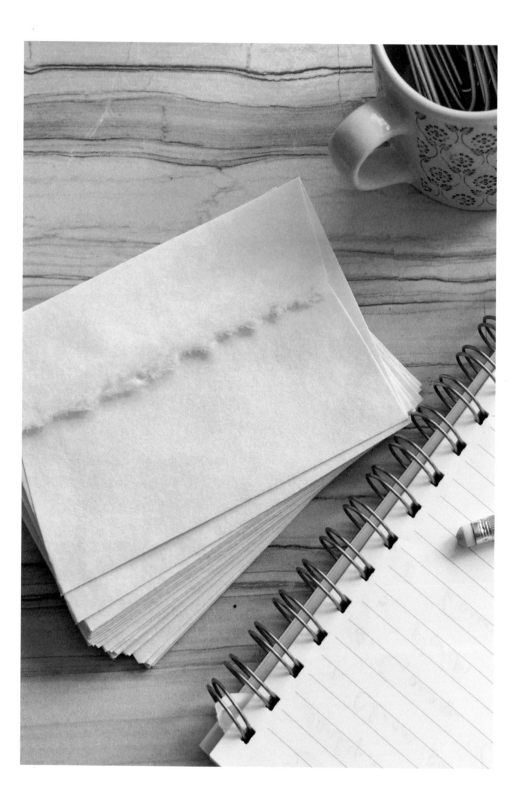

3

DECISIONS

.

TO KEEP OR NOT TO KEEP; THAT IS THE DECISION.

.

Your decision. This is where our story begins.
And – spoiler alert – where it will end too.
Everything you are about to do hinges on
developing the skill of decision-making.
Are you ready?

First, let's try to figure out where the
disorganisation and clutter comes from and why
it's so hard to make decisions about it.

.

Clutter is anything you no longer use, need or love. *Clutter is caused by deferred decision-making.*

The reason for putting off decisions is the other things going on in your life. Clutter is merely the symptom, not the cause. Clutter is not just a load of stuff, not just physical things we can touch. It can also be:

- ✓ **BAD HABITS**
- ✓ **DISTRACTIONS**
- ✓ **SAYING YES WHEN YOU WANT TO SAY NO**
- ✓ **SAYING NO WHEN YOU WANT TO SAY YES**
- ✓ **OVER-BOOKING YOUR CHILDREN**
- ✓ **BEING UNDER-PREPARED FOR A MEETING**

Which of those do you no longer use, need or love having in your life?

Every client I work with has some clutter to deal with. After an hour or so, I'm asked the same question: 'Am I the worst you've worked with?' Everyone is mortified by their clutter. We feel shame, feel we are not on top of things the way we 'should' be, embarrassed because we feel we 'should' be able to tidy our home without hired help.

Clutter leads us down the path of comparison. We feel inadequate because we think everyone else has life all figured out. A cluttered home makes us feel we're not coping, we're not a good partner or parent. We compare ourselves to others and think they are better at tidying, more productive and generally more equipped to cope. No one has as much clutter in their lives as you. There's embarrassment too. You give up inviting friends over and, worse, you won't allow the kids to bring friends home.

You get embarrassed at the thought of an Organiser going through your delicates or parking outside your home with a sign on their car advertising to the neighbourhood that you have clutter.

It comes back to good old parochial mindset. The attempt to keep up with the Joneses and being mindful of what the neighbours think.

PROCRASTINATION

If clutter is the symptom, procrastination is the cause. Procrastination is, and always will be, the enemy of organisation. You can't fix one without fixing the other. How many times a day do you think, 'I'll just leave this here for now' or 'I'll come back to that in a minute'?

In that moment you have chosen not to put something away. You have something in your hand, and you either don't know what to do with it and have no intention of figuring that out now, or you're running out of time, so you put it down and move on. You choose not to make a decision on it. You choose not to make it a priority. When you do this often enough, clutter builds up.

In *The Organized Mind*, Daniel Levitin says, 'if our self-confidence and the value of completing the task are both high, we're less likely to procrastinate' (Levitin p.198).

This is exactly why you are not organising your home or workplace. You don't think it's that big a deal to put something off for just a bit longer. You can't see the value in organising and therefore aren't encouraged to change a behaviour. Even if you did try to get organised, you feel you can't do it well enough and even if you could, you doubt it would last, so why bother?

Time after time, you feel that you don't have time to make a decision about something, so you put off dealing with it. What you need to realise is that you *have* made a decision. You've made a decision not to make a decision. *You've decided to not deal with it.* That decision will have a consequence: perhaps losing something important; losing time; having an argument; over-extending yourself; stress. Worse still, when it all comes to a head and the straw breaks the camel's back, you will be suffering from such a massive sense of being overwhelmed that you won't know what to do or where to start. Which leads to another cycle of procrastination.

We procrastinate because of the emotions that decisions bring up. Here are some of the main reasons why people keep things.

'But it cost a fortune'

This is one of the top reasons people give me for keeping things. This one makes us feel guilty. We feel awful that we wasted our money on this item and then never used it. We keep it, just in case we might get our money's worth out of it.

In reality, the expensive pair of shoes make your feet sore, the dress is too small, the shirt was an impulse buy and you don't even like it. But they are left to gather dust and we think, 'I'll get rid of it next time.'

The reason why this item stays is because it cost money. But the real reason is that it makes us feel guilty and we decide not to deal with that. We are afraid of losing the money we spent on it.

Whether you give it away or keep it and leave it at the back of your cupboard, you've still lost your money. Either use it or let it go.

'I feel awful giving it away'

When we're decluttering we often come across items that have been given to us by a kind-hearted family member or friend. We think, 'It was really kind of them to give us the stroller when the baby was two weeks old, even though we'd already bought our own, but I just feel we should keep it.'

We do it to them too. We might have a dress or a toy or a handbag that we don't need and we think our sister or mother or friend will use it, so we give it to them.

Our excuse is 'I should keep it because X gave it to me,' but the real reason is that we feel guilty about not using it and guilty about giving it away. Or we're afraid they'll find out we gave it away and would be disappointed. Those awkward feelings stop us making a decision about whether or not we actually want it.

Sentimental items are the hardest of all to declutter. All the little things that spark a memory. Your child's first tooth, his first drawing or school report; concert tickets; engagement cards; itineraries from an amazing holiday. We have so much memorabilia and that is lovely to keep. Unfortunately, though, the feelings connected with some items sometimes lead people to keep everything.

Keeping your child's artwork is a lovely thing to do, but you don't need every piece they made. They will enjoy looking over their pictures when they're grown up, but they won't want to look over all of them. Holding on to some family heirlooms is important for the family history. But your children will not appreciate every single ornament or document. They will only have to declutter it themselves one day. And if you keep too much, it will make it difficult for them to know the genuinely important items to save. Keep the items that are the real treasures.

Sentimentality can make getting rid of some items very difficult. Be mindful as to what excuses you are using to keep an item. Are these excuses good enough, or is sadness or fear making you defer the decision again? If you consider everything 'precious', then nothing really is.

It surprises me how much rubbish is left around a house. I feel so sad when I see plastic, empty packaging and cardboard that should have been thrown out ages ago lying around a house. The clutter has taken so much control that even rubbish has been given permission to take up space in a home.

The idea that organised people can't be creative and creative people are naturally messy really gets under my skin. It is a myth, and it irritates me because that sort of thinking made me believe it about myself. I never thought I could be a creative person. I was hopeless at crafts, I didn't have the patience to plait my hair, I make a mess whenever I paint my nails and I can only cook basic dinners. But I've come to realise that the organisation I put into my house and my clients' homes comes from my creativity. I can arrange items to make them look beautiful; I know how to make a room function better just by looking at it. Every person is creative in different ways; creativity isn't just an ability to draw, write, dance, sing. And disorganisation and creativity aren't linked.

Creativity is within us. Tidying up does not remove your creativity or dampen your artistic soul. Neither does a mess. In my opinion, clutter slows down your opportunities to be creative, but creativity is always there. Like air. Mess or no mess.

CLUTTER SLOWS DOWN YOUR OPPORTUNITIES TO BE CREATIVE.

Let's look at some more specific items you may struggle with:

SITUATION	EMOTION/ WHY	DECISION	ACTION	RESULT	THOUGHTS
BABY CLOTHES	Guilt – of a child lost Sadness – not having more children/that they're grown up	'I'll come back to it'	Leaves clothes in attic	Attic becomes full	'I'll never get a handle on this' 'I can't do anything right'
CLOTHES	Sadness, regret, guilt – from divorce/ break-up/ gained weight	'I won't throw it out because I might fit into it again' 'What if he comes back?'	Leaves clothes in wardrobe	Wardrobe becomes full	'It's always a mess' 'So is the whole house'
TOYS	Guilt – not being home more, sick/ disabled child Love/need – to give them what you didn't have Resentment – under pressure to tidy up	'I'll have to ask them before I get rid of it' 'They'll notice if I throw that out'	Toys remain	Toy room becomes full	'They've too much stuff' 'I'm living in a play room' 'I don't want to clear this on my weekend off' 'I can't maintain it, so why bother?'
PAPERWORK	Fear – of what you'll find/that you'll make a mistake dealing with it	'I'll wait until my partner can help me with it; we'll do it together'	Papers are left on kitchen counter, couch, beside the bed	Paperwork is scattered in multiple areas of the home Important documents can't be found when needed	'I don't know where to start' 'I'm just a disorganised person'

As you can see, we make a lot of excuses about why we don't get rid of items and why we don't organise. Underneath every excuse is a real emotionally charged reason. We keep items because of how the decision to let them go makes us *feel*. Even though these items don't make us feel good, we don't use them and we don't enjoy them, they stay in our home because getting rid of them makes us feel even worse. We feel guilty, emotional, overwhelmed, stressed, powerless at the prospect. So of course, we don't make a decision. We say, 'I'll leave it there for now' or, 'I'll come back to it' or, 'It's fine there for the moment.'

Unfortunately, our things tend to accumulate. The emotion that caused you to keep something in the first place is one thing, but as clutter builds, you look at the entire situation and catastrophise it. Now it's not about one particular item; it's about the whole room, the whole house and, worse, your ability.

WHAT'S HAPPENING IN YOUR BRAIN?

To understand this better, I had a crash course in brain anatomy from Dr Keane.

The brain is made up of three layers. First the spinal cord and brain stem. This is what keeps us alive. Then there's the limbic system, which is responsible for our emotions and moods. The layer we think of as 'the brain' is the neocortex layer, which deals with higher-order functions, including decision-making. If we make decisions that are linked to an emotion, this triggers the limbic system.

'If you get emotional about things, the ability of the neocortex becomes less efficient because emotions have exceptional power. The emotional part of the brain is looking for easy solutions,' explains Dr Keane.

Limbic system trumps neocortex. Emotion trumps logic. Heart trumps head.

FEAR

Does it come down to fear? Everything in life boils down to a decision, a balancing act between choice and risk. You might make the right decision, but then again you might make the wrong one. Uncertainty is a scary feeling.

In her book *Big Magic*, Elizabeth Gilbert discusses fear in relation to her writing. She imagines fear as a passenger with her on a road trip. Fear, she suggests, can come along for the drive if it wants, but it won't be allowed to touch the maps, the radio, suggest detours, and 'above all else, my dear old familiar friend, you are absolutely forbidden to drive' (Gilbert, p. 26).

As you declutter, your body will recoil and your head will tell you that you aren't decluttering right or you're making a mistake. That's fear of uncertainty around the decisions you're making.

Some items can stir strong emotions in us. It's when strong emotions arise that organising becomes overwhelming. The thought of making a decision on these items causes real confusion and sometimes anxiety.

✓ 'I'LL KEEP IT, JUST IN CASE I NEED IT SOMEDAY.'

✓ 'IT MIGHT COME BACK INTO FASHION.'

✓ 'I DON'T HAVE ENOUGH OF IT.'

✓ 'SOMEONE ELSE IN THE FAMILY MIGHT USE IT.'

✓ 'I ACTUALLY DO HAVE A HOME FOR IT UPSTAIRS.'

✓ 'I'D BETTER CHECK WITH MY OTHER HALF FIRST.'

✓ 'THE KIDS WOULD NOTICE IF I GOT RID OF IT.'

I've heard it all. I've seen the struggles. My clients say everything except the one thing that's hurting the most: *'I won't make this decision now just in case I regret it.'*

Sometimes it helps to ask yourself: 'What if I do regret the decision? What's the worst thing that can happen?' If an item is too tricky to deal with right now, come back to it. Often it's much easier to make a decision on it with a second look later on. Only you can weigh up the implications for your life and home space of keeping something or letting it go.

Becoming organised requires a change of thought and a change of approach. Swap negative thoughts for more positive ones.

PERFECTIONISM

My clients often think that my home never gets messy. But of course it does. And I don't always fold my pyjamas, I don't like spending my Saturday cleaning my home, I do run late for appointments and my car could be left unwashed for six months. For me, organisation is about comfort, not perfection. *Perfectionism is not a comfortable state because it is unachievable.*

That's not to say I don't suffer from perfectionism sometimes, but I do recognise when I'm prone to it. The more stressed I feel, the more 'perfect' I want things to be. That's a need for control in a situation where I feel out of control. It can also come from tiredness and feeling overwhelmed.

So there is the assumption that organised people are perfectionists. But there are varying degrees of 'perfectionism'.

In her book *Daring Greatly*, Brené Brown explains perfectionism as 'self-destructive simply because perfection doesn't exist. It's an unattainable goal. Perfectionism is more about perception than internal motivation, and there is no way to control perception ... if we want freedom from perfectionism, we have to make the long journey from "what will people think?" to "I am enough"' (Brown, pp.130–1).

But disorganised people are perfectionists too.

Wait, what?

Well, for sure! Perfectionism stops many people starting projects. Perfectionism also stops projects from ever being finished. Perfectionists won't start anything unless they can do it right. They need the perfect time, the perfect storage, the perfect help. Which never materialises. As a result, their projects are put off. They procrastinate. Alternatively, too much time is spent on one task over another. Deadlines are missed and energy is drained.

Many people with clutter in their space, and in their schedules, are perfectionists too.

What can we do to help make decisions when it comes to organising?

ACCEPTING 'GOOD ENOUGH'

One solution is getting comfortable with being 'good enough'. With organisation being 'good enough', with projects being 'good enough'. Organised people are very aware of their time and therefore prioritise. Prioritising allows tasks to get done well enough. First find the solution that's good enough. If you want, and have the time, you can always perfect it later.

I said earlier that I can leave my car unwashed for six months. Does a dirty car irritate me? Sure! But not enough to choose to do something about it over something more important. I'll get to it when I have time.

In organising sessions, clients sometimes get ahead of themselves. We could be working in the living room and we'll start with the TV console. We'll get that done and move to the china cabinet. While we're working on the cabinet, the client realises that we only have another hour left in the session and we still have to finish the cabinet and move to the bookshelves. In an attempt to get to the goal of 'being organised', a client will often jump ahead and start taking books off the shelves. They think that the living room won't be organised unless the bookshelves are sorted. As energy starts to lag, panic rears its ugly head and causes the client to force the process.

However, accepting good enough and staying in the present moment are key when decluttering.

It may well be that by the end of the session, the bookshelves still need to be done. However, the rest of the room will look great. The bookshelves probably won't take all that long and can be done quickly at the start of the next session and then we'll move on to the next room.

By jumping ahead, the client makes things harder on him/herself. More and more clutter has just been added to an area that was almost done! The bookshelves may be clear, but now everything is on the floor. In an attempt to get to the final goal, the client wants to clear space, which is totally understandable.

However, as we will see in the next chapter, it would never have worked from a time point of view. All the morning's work would have come undone just for a *feeling* that we were getting closer to a goal. In fact, we were closer to the goal before emptying the bookshelves because the work was being done in a systematic way.

But that's why I'm here! I totally understand it, so I'll jump in and stop the panic. Let's stay in the present moment, declutter and organise where we are and let's not worry about the rest of it just right now. Recognise partial wins and accept 'good enough' for today. You can perfect it later when time allows. That's where balance comes in. Be aware of what has pushed you over into discomfort and into feeling overwhelmed.

Brené Brown says that her research participants explained that reducing their anxiety involved 'paying attention to how much they could do and how much was too much, and learning how to say "enough"' (Brown, p.142).

What is your limit? What allows you to live and work productively and what happens in your environment to push you into being overwhelmed?

CATEGORISATION AND SYSTEMS

Organising at its most basic level is categorising. Organised people are always categorising what they own and the time they have.

Daniel Levitin, in *The Organized Mind*, discusses our brains as energy economisers and categorisers. 'The act of categorizing helps us to organise the physical world-out-there but also organises the mental world, the world-in-here, in our heads and thus what we can pay attention to and remember' (Levitin, p. 22).

He goes on: 'the most fundamental principle of the organized mind, the one most critical to keeping us from forgetting or losing things, is to *shift the burden of organizing from our brains to the external world* … the information you need is in the physical pile there not crowded in your head up here. Successful people have devised dozens of ways to do this, physical reminders in their homes, cars, offices and throughout their lives to shift the burden of remembering from their brains to their environment' (Levitin, p. 35)

And this is the absolute crux of it. This is how and why we organise.

Let's look at this a bit more closely. The average person has more possessions than ever before. Combine that with everything we have to do: raise children, clean the house, go to work, organise travel, do the shopping, and so on and so on. Our brain has to keep track of all these things. Our possessions are increasing, what we have to do is increasing, information is increasing; but we seem to have less time to do it all.

In Chapter 1 we discussed how when life throws us a curveball it brings many different things into perspective. Unexpected events need brain space and brain power. They require decisions and often involve a lot of emotion.

Therefore, the more systems you can create in your life, by organising your physical space and what you own, managing your time, prioritising and creating routines, the less your brain has to remember. It is therefore free to think about larger stressors in your life if and when it needs.

Olympic athletes like Michael Phelps visualise their morning before a competition so that they know exactly what is going to happen before it happens. Former President Barack Obama and Facebook CEO Mark Zuckerberg wear a limited range of clothes so that they don't have to think about what to wear.

The more we can categorise our time and our things into systems in our external environment, the less stressed we feel. We reduce neural fatigue and minimise complexity in our life. We shift the burden of remembering from our brain to our external world. This increases our ability to focus on what we need to focus on.

BEING MINDFUL

Imagine that you're clearing the kitchen table or island. You find some items belonging to your daughter, so you take them to her room. In her room the curtains are still shut and the bed isn't made, so you go about fixing that. Then the phone rings and this delays you for another 10 minutes before you finally make it back to the kitchen.

Or you arrive home from food shopping and put all the freezer food away, but everything else is left on the floor. Or you empty the car for the annual car service and a week later the items are still sitting in your hallway.

Some of us lack focus. Our attention wanders and we get distracted. Therefore we need to practise more mindfulness. We can train the brain to focus just that little bit more. Having systems or a 'home' for everything is part of that training. If we make a conscious effort to reduce what we own and to create a good way of storing what we have, it is easier to focus when we put things down and put things away. Being more mindful about how we treat our stuff and how we treat our space becomes a habit.

CHANGING THE HABITS OF A LIFETIME

In order to get yourself and your home organised you need to declutter. In order to see a real difference, we need to acknowledge that any decent organising is going to involve making a decision and understanding our emotions.

Making a D-ecision + Understanding our E-motions = D.E. Clutter

Getting organised involves creating systems. This in turn involves making decisions that in some cases may challenge our emotions. That is why we 'become organised', we don't simply 'get organised'. The disorganisation and clutter didn't build up overnight and it's not going to go overnight either. *Becoming organised is* a process of changing a certain lifestyle and *becoming more aware of our stuff, our space, our time and ourselves.*

In *The Power of Habit*, Charles Duhigg says that 'to modify a habit, you must decide to change it' (Duhigg 2013, p. 270). The more decisions we make, the more in control we feel. The more in control we feel, the more motivated we become. The more motivated we become, the more decisions we can make. It's cyclical.

When you are feeling overwhelmed, it is the decision to take action that starts the change. Taking any action, no matter how small, gives you power.

It all starts with ourselves: understanding why we do what we do and learning how to change our behaviour. Then we put new habits into practice.

The journey of becoming organised starts and ends with yourself. You learn about what you own and why you keep it, how you'd like to store it and why it's important for your current home or work life. You have a certain personality, a certain way of living, and your stuff and your space will be affected. Will your stuff and space enhance your life or control it? That's your decision.

In the next few chapters I will show you how to create systems in your schedule and space in order to facilitate your new habits. Then we'll come back to the self and examine routines that will solidify these habits.

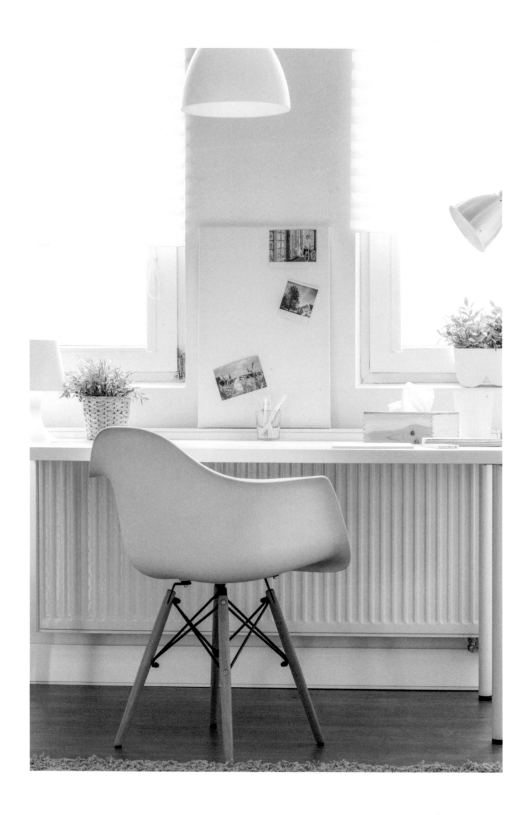

4

GOALS

.

SO NOW WE KNOW THE BENEFITS OF
BECOMING ORGANISED AND WHY IT CAN
BE HARD TO GET STARTED.

.

But get started we must. And to kick-start it all,
we need to figure out why you're doing any
of this in the first place. Why would someone
voluntarily take hours out of their already busy
day to organise themselves, or get someone to
help them organise?

.

We know that we've reached the point where we need to do something.

We also know that relief can give us false hope. We need to know our long-term goals so that when the pain starts to subside and you start to see a result, you're encouraged to keep going to the end, not give up halfway through.

Organising is non-urgent, so it's low on your list of priorities. The irony, of course, is that if you take time out to do this work, many things in your life will go from urgent to non-urgent. Therefore, in order to get started and to keep it up you have to know *why* you're doing it.

Every decision we make is ours. We can ask advice, ask for help, speak to a therapist. But ultimately, we always have a choice. Even if someone else makes the decision for us, we have to make the decision to allow them to do so.

That's why it's so important to have an idea of your bigger picture. Whether that's a goal, resolution, personal value, if you know *why* you are doing or not doing something, and what you are hoping to achieve, it makes all your decisions that little bit easier.

An entrepreneur who's convinced of the value of his business will live on beans and toast to put all his money into the business. A mother will suffer the sadness of letting go of boxes of baby clothes so that she can create and organise a new office and explore a different life from the one she thought she'd have.

These are 'bigger picture' goals. What are yours? What's really important to you? What happened to make you feel you need to get organised? And what is in your future that you think being organised is going to help? *How would being more organised make you feel*, do you think?

Write down how you think you will feel without clutter. This will help you get to the heart of *why* you want to declutter.

And it's not just about getting organised. Your personal *why* can determine whether you say yes or no to moving to another country, say yes or no to staying with your partner, say yes or no to leaving a permanent job and starting a business, saying yes or no to staying in bed late.

These are the bigger reasons why you will dedicate several sessions to clearing a spare room, attic or garage. They are the goals driven by emotion.

Getting comfortable with uncertainty, and linking the tasks you have to do with a goal you want, provide the focus and motivation you need and makes decisions more manageable.

VISUALISE

Now you know why you are organising, but what will it look like? Let's say your big picture goal is to clear the spare room in order to create an office for your new business. Or maybe you've saved enough money for a new kitchen and you want it to be clutter-free from day one. Your goals are great, but what will the spare room or the kitchen actually look like?

This is the fun part! Imagine your dream office, or your dream garage, or your dream kitchen. What kind of organisation would you like to see? What labelling do you like? What gorgeous products could you use? What colours and furniture do you like?

Create a mood board of images that you like. Begin to look at the aesthetics, style, era and colours you are attracted to. Use magazines, brochures and newspapers to cut out pictures you like. Or do it online through Pinterest and Houzz and discover your inner creativity and what you love. If you can visualise it, you increase your chances of making it a reality. The vision of what you want to achieve will help keep you motivated when times get tough.

OTHER ASPECTS OF YOUR LIFE

As you declutter and start to clear space, the benefits will flow into other areas of your life. You will feel lighter, more in control, and you will have more time. You will be thinking more clearly, so you can consider doing things you hadn't the physical or mental energy to do before. So what would you like to do with this additional space in your schedule? Start dating? Take up an art class? Take the kids swimming every week? Travel? Start a blog? Or perhaps you might find the strength to give up something?

Look at the other areas of your life that you feel need attention. Let your subconscious work on these areas too as you are physically shifting clutter and making space.

- ✓ **RELATIONSHIPS**
- ✓ **WORK/BUSINESS**
- ✓ **HEALTH**
- ✓ **INTERESTS**
- ✓ **COMMUNITY**
- ✓ **SPIRITUAL**
- ✓ **FINANCE**

To ease you in gently, try these questions, write down your answers and see how you feel afterwards.

- If my home was organised, I would feel...
  (Keep this positive. For example, 'calmer' rather than 'less anxious'.)

- If my home was organised, I would do...
  (Is there anything you've been thinking you'd like to do, but feel you don't have the time?)

- If my home was organised, my home would look...
  (Close your eyes and visualise your home. What colours and images come to mind?)

EXPECTATIONS

People often tell me that they love the minimalist look. I'm actually surprised how often I hear it. However, this is a knee-jerk reaction to too much clutter. They are surrounded by so much stuff that they want to go to the opposite extreme.

It takes a lot of work, and even more discipline, to achieve minimalism. If you have a lot of clutter, a busy life and a few kids, the chances are that this is an unrealistic goal. And probably one you don't really want anyway. Knowing what you want and what your goals are is so important to stop you going from one extreme to the other and then getting disappointed and demotivated.

So keep your expectations of yourself, your space and those you share the space with in check. If we understand why we do things, how we can change and have an end goal in sight, all we need now is the time to actually do the work and put it all into practice.

Without better scheduling you can't save your space. So let's do just that and find some time for you in your schedule.

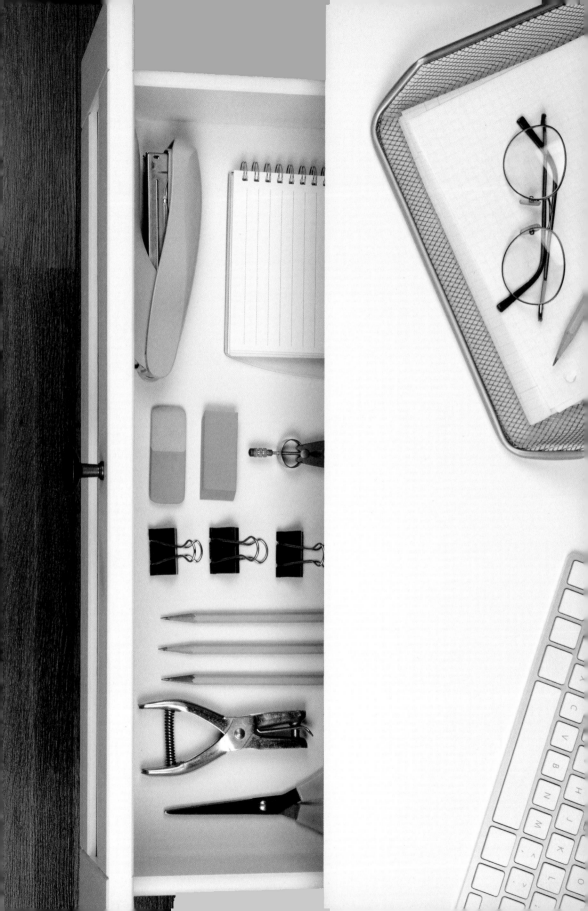

Part II

Your Schedule

·

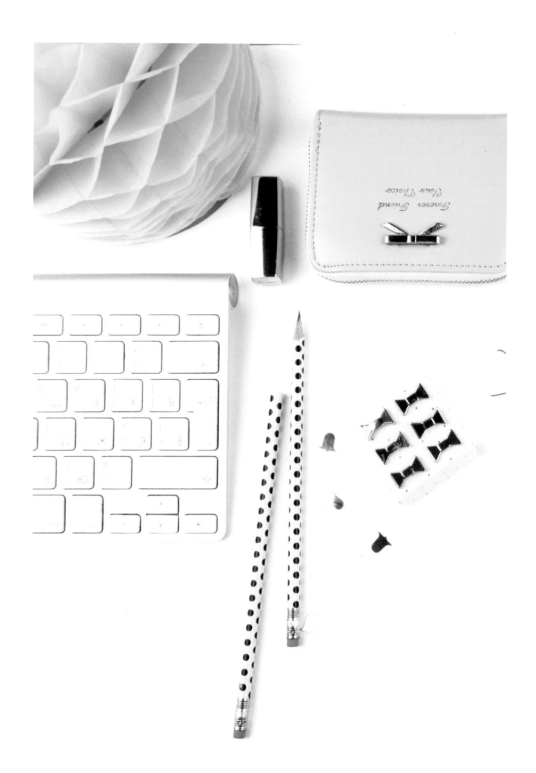

5

LIST IT

·

YOU CANNOT ORGANISE YOUR HOME WITHOUT EXAMINING YOUR RELATIONSHIP WITH TIME.

·

Disorganisation and poor time management go hand in hand. As the American entrepreneur Jim Rohn said, '*Either you run the day, or the day runs you.*' In the same way, if you don't control clutter, it will control you. As we saw in Chapter 2, decluttering and organising is non-urgent. There are plenty of other things we'd rather do with our day than sort paper, clothes and toys. It's very easy to consistently push it down our priority list. Too easy not to bother.

·

Therefore, if we're going to declutter, the time period we require had better jump out at us waving frantically and screaming 'Pick me, pick me! You have nothing else to do!' Chances of this happening? Slim, very slim – unless you know exactly how all your time and all your other priorities are mapped out. When you know the time you have available and how you use it, as well as your tasks and their priority levels, then, and only then, can you allocate slots of time to decluttering. And other non-urgent tasks, for that matter.

Clutter has built up over time and you need time to shift it. The amount of time you need to give it depends on the amount of clutter and disorganisation you're dealing with and what result you want. You have to make time to do it, but this is often easier said than done.

How do you find this time of which I speak? Consider the three Ls:

✓ **LIST IT**   ✓ **LOG IT**   ✓ **LAY IT OUT**

Write your lists, log your time and lay out this information in a schedule.

Let's start with a list. Most people have written a list of things they need to get done. Some people, like myself, do this regularly. Some people love lists; others loathe them.

I, of course, think they work. Now, I don't necessarily manage to tick off everything on my list, but what I love about a list is that it gets things out of my head. Life is very busy and every day is filled with things I have to do for the family, the house, work, friends and myself. Having that all jumping around my subconscious is just not for me. So I write a list. This lightens my mental load. Seeing everything written down allows me to distinguish the important stuff from the not-so-important stuff. When I can do that, I can plan and prioritise. The very act of writing the list helps me focus on the things that require my attention.

MASTER TO-DO LISTS

A Master to-do list is for your short- to medium-term to-dos. These are the tasks that are hurtling towards you every day, week and month, so fast that many of them remain unticked!

The Master List is getting everything written down and out of your head – calming the hamster in the wheel. That's all it is.

HOME VS WORK

I suggest splitting the Master List into Home and Work. Then you can see at a glance what you need to do in both 'lives'. It will help you schedule your work so that you get more time at home, and it will allow you to slot some personal tasks into your work day – such as 'schedule the dentist' or 'sign school notes'. Here's a sample Master List.

MASTER LIST

HOME	WORK
Pay TV licence	Pay web designer
Buy Clare a gift for baby	Ring last week's client
Ring around for new car insurance policy	Back up computer files
Order school uniform	Update August social media
Buy Hannah's shoes	Sign off on next month's marketing campaign
Call phone company regarding contract	Call John R
Sort summer/winter clothes	Email re: advertisement
Send Jamie's birthday card	Order business cards
Book restaurant for Friday night	Photocopy notes for Thursday's meeting

PAPERWORK

A lot of the tasks on this list are going to be created by paperwork. As you go through paperwork in Chapter 17, you will find bills to pay, Post-its with phone numbers to ring, insurance companies you need to email. All that paperwork is left out to remind you to get a task done. However, simply leaving it out doesn't get the job done. Scheduling it does.

Start writing the Master List by thinking of your most pressing tasks. Get those out of your head. Once that's done, look around your home or office at the loose paper lying around. Go through the paperwork, and add the task that each piece of paper creates to the Master List under the relevant column. An invoice from your web designer goes under 'work', a TV licence bill goes under 'home'. Keep the paper to one side. (If you can do this step, that is – you may have too much paperwork, in which case wait until Chapter 17.)

Now we have a list of tasks and we will make time to get them done.

Keep the Master List to hand for the next few hours. Now that your mind has started to empty, more things to deal with will come to the fore and you will want to catch them quickly.

And remember. One list. It could be several pages – if so, staple them together – but stick to that one document. If you wish to do it digitally, by all means do so. I personally think the physical act of writing the Master List is more helpful. After that, when you start to do daily lists you can switch to digital.

It might be overwhelming to have seven A4 pages full of to-dos, just as it's overwhelming to look at your house and find clutter in every room. But this is an act of staying in the present moment. It's sitting with the discomfort. It is what it is.

The good news? Most of what's on that Master List you won't even bother with. So relax. We'll worry about the contents later. Right now, it's just an act of writing. *Start emptying your head.*

DAILY TO-DO LISTS

Once you have created your Master to-do list you can use it to create your Daily to-do lists.

By referring to your Master List, you can take tasks from there and add them to your Daily Lists. That will help you get things done!

Every evening, write your to-do list for tomorrow. You could make one list of tasks or split the Daily List by home and work as you did with the Master List. Each day, pull items off the Master List and add them to your Daily List.

You will be able to do this more effectively when you start to add schedules, but you can get started now. One of the most important things to remember when you are adding tasks to your to-do list is to think about exactly what each task involves. Let's look at breaking down tasks.

Every job, task, project you need to do can be broken down into a beginning, middle and end. I imagine each task as a circle that has to be closed to complete the task.

When you have something to do, think about everything you need to get it finished. Any to-do usually includes other little jobs you need to do to get the task done. For example, you write on your to-do list, 'Organise Oliver's birthday party'. But your scheduling of this task won't work if you leave it at that. You have to be specific. What does organising the party actually involve?

You need to list all the elements, for example:

✓ ORDER BIRTHDAY CAKE

✓ COLLECT BIRTHDAY CAKE

✓ BUY CANDLES

✓ BUY GIFT AND CARD

✓ BUY DECORATIONS

✓ CREATE INVITATIONS

✓ POST/DELIVER INVITATIONS

✓ CONFIRM ATTENDEES

✓ CLEAN THE HOUSE

Or you write on your to-do list, 'Get shelving for toy room'. But that job actually involves a trip to the suppliers and everything that goes along with that.

✓ **TAKE MEASUREMENTS OF THE WALL**

✓ **WRITE OUT SHOPPING LIST OF OTHER ITEMS I NEED**

✓ **GO TO SUPPLIERS**

✓ **ORGANISE DELIVERY OF PURCHASES**

✓ **BUILD SHELVING**

✓ **ORGANISE TOYS ON SHELVING**

We can break it down even further:

✓ **PREPARATION**
Take measurements of the wall
Write out shopping list of other items I need

✓ **TASK**
Go to suppliers
Organise delivery of purchases
Build shelving
Organise toys on shelving

✓ **CLEAR-UP**
Dispose of packaging
Return any unused purchases

Most people do the preparation before a task but don't bother with clearing up until much later. They want to get on to the next job, then the job after that, leaving clutter in their wake. Getting the task done can be difficult enough, but once the task is over we're often so relieved that we collapse and relax or we have to push on to the next thing.

It's very important to close the circle. *Finish the job at hand.* If you don't it will nag away at you, creating mind clutter. The work is not done until it is done.

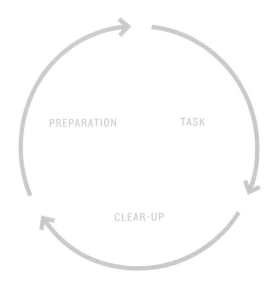

PREPARATION   TASK

CLEAR-UP

Have a look at these scenarios. Do any of them ring a bell?

1   **YOUR CHILD IS GOING TO A BIRTHDAY PARTY AND YOU'RE WRAPPING THE GIFT.** Once that's done, you're out the door, leaving the scissors, tape, and paper wrapping remains on the table.

2   **THE KIDS ARRIVE HOME ON THEIR LAST DAY OF SCHOOL BEFORE THE SUMMER HOLIDAYS.** They have an armful of artwork and projects from the last year. In the excitement, everything is dumped in the nearest available space. As the summer months pass, this paper, art and craftwork circulate over the surfaces of your home. When September arrives you feel so guilty that you never looked through it that, once again, you don't do anything with it. You leave the artwork in a pile and swear you'll get to it this week.

3   **THE KIDS ARE DOING THEIR HOMEWORK ON THE KITCHEN TABLE.** Dinner is ready, so homework and school supplies are pushed to one side. Next morning, everyone scrambles looking for copies, notes and pencil cases.

All of these scenarios involve procrastination. In each scenario there is a decision to not complete the circle of the task.

The gift wrap is not put back in a drawer. The school work is scattered in numerous places and precious art work that might be lovely to keep gets crumpled at the bottom of a school bag. Or maybe the suitcase is not emptied after a holiday or the dinner dishes are loaded into the dishwasher but the pots and pans are left at the sink.

Clear-up finishes the immediate task at hand. This may be a stand-alone task or it may form part of a longer-term project, but the process is the same. For example, look at the tasks below. Some are short; others will take longer.

TASK	PREPARATION	CLEAR-UP
Weekly shop	Write shopping list	Empty bags, put bags away
Go to work	Organise bag, make lunch, get clothes ready	Clean lunch box, hang up coat
Renovating a house	Meetings, permissions, research, design	Empty moving boxes, file all documentation

The duration of the tasks varies. Your weekly shop might take 30 minutes. Renovating a house could take six months. But they all require clear-up at the end to finish them.

As we will see with organising our space, we always want to set up items for their next use. The same is true of tasks. If the job at hand is part of a project that you will have to revisit over and over again for the next few weeks, you need to be able to pick up where you left off.

For that to happen, you need to clear up the last bit of work you did each time, whether it's putting the shopping bags away or labelling and filing a folder. This means that next time you need to go food shopping the bags are waiting for you. Next time you are meeting your architect, you know where to find the plans. You know exactly where you left off with a task and you won't be wasting time and energy reviewing what you did last time or searching for an item before you can get on with today's task.

The problem is that people think clear-up is going to take ages, which is why it's left on the long finger. The only clear-up that takes ages is the clear-up that wasn't done at the time of the task or shortly after. Unfinished clear-up results in clutter and needs a much larger bank of time to sort through.

Any clear-up you can't do there and then needs to be bumped up the priority list and slotted in to be done as soon as possible. This is because it is so much quicker to finish off a task when you're in it than to do it later.

'Later' results in procrastination. As the day progresses, more to-dos will be on your radar, more information will come into your day. Therefore, anything not done at the time of the task is added to more and more uncompleted tasks, which means more and more clear-up time and less and less time for you.

Remember this mantra:

✓ **PREPARATION**

✓ **TASK**

✓ **CLEAR UP**

✓ **MOVE ON**

If you don't have a realistic idea of what is involved in the tasks you need to do, you won't be realistic about the time you need to get the work done.

In the next chapter we'll look at logging the time it takes for tasks and breaking them down. Before that, let's make your to-do list work for you.

Once tasks are added to the to-do list, many people stop there. However, we want to make the list earn its keep. There are several ways to do this: prioritising and grouping tasks are two of the best.

PRIORITISING

This is the single most important skill to learn when you are trying to become more organised.

Time management is a constant juggling act with your priorities. Some of these are urgent and stress-inducing; others are enjoyable and life-enhancing. We are constantly trying to balance them. Prioritising identifies what's important to us in relation to our values and goals, and we prioritise tasks by comparing their worth.

IT IS MUCH
QUICKER TO
FINISH OFF A
TASK WHEN
YOU ARE IN IT
THAN TO DO
IT LATER.

We are constantly searching for more time, saying almost daily, 'I don't have time!' But time management expert Laura Vanderkam said in her TED talk, 'How to Gain Control of your Free Time', that 'it's not that we don't have time to do something, it's that it's not a priority for us'.

This was a real 'a-ha!' moment for me. How true it is! We always have time for what we deem to be important to us. We can't say we don't have time for something if we choose to do one thing when we know that another one is more important.

Stephen Covey suggests in his book *The 7 Habits of Highly Effective People* that our 'challenge is not to manage time, but to manage ourselves' (Covey, p.150). He uses the Time Management Matrix to show that we spend our time in one of four ways. Any task you need to do usually falls into one of the quadrants: important and urgent; important but not urgent; not important but urgent; not important and not urgent.

You can't ignore anything urgent, whether it's important or not. However, the more organised you become, the fewer urgent tasks you have. Important but not urgent, Covey says, is 'the heart of effective personal management' (Covey p.153). This is where you carry out tasks that develop your business goals, relationship goals, fitness goals, etc. Unfortunately, procrastination leads us to spend a lot of time on tasks that are not important or urgent. We think we're getting things done, and we are, but unfortunately not the tasks that are going to make a difference in our lives.

For example, how many of us log onto our phones and spend 30 minutes on social media without even realising it? Or we watch television instead of getting ourselves ready for tomorrow's meeting? Or our ankle twinges slightly and it's enough to avoid exercise class this week?

We've created the Master List, and our Daily Lists are created from that. Now we need to identify the most important and/or urgent tasks on those lists.

Start by numbering each task. Your number one task is top priority. This is either an urgent task or non–urgent but important. It may be a task that would make a real difference to your workload or your home space but you keep putting it off. It could be anything from arranging insurance for your car to identifying all the art and photographs you want to hang up and calling the handyman to book him in.

As Mark Twain wrote, 'If it's your job to eat a frog, it's best to do it first thing in the morning. And if it's your job to eat two frogs, it's best to eat the biggest one first.' In other words, do the worst or the most difficult jobs first and get them over with. They are the totally unappealing tasks that will make you feel really good when they're done or will produce the results you really need in your home or work life. Or both!

You can assign a priority number to tasks that are enjoyable and fun and are neither important nor urgent. For instance, 'post birthday card' is an easy task, so you might give it a low priority number of 6. You will get around to posting the birthday card, but the point of prioritising is that it prevents you spending time dealing with task 6 when task 1 is still outstanding.

Prioritising takes a lot of discipline, particularly at the start. If you are feeling disorganised and out of control, getting clear about what's a priority and what's not and taking the relevant action will move you towards a more organised feeling.

GROUPING TASKS

Identifying your priorities is the most important thing you can do to make your to-do list work and get tasks moved off it. Once you know what your priorities are, you can also group tasks.

By location

If you have to leave the house or office, think about what else you could get done while you're out. For example, buy stamps while you're out food shopping, or lodge a cheque in the bank on your way to a meeting. If you have an appointment on the high street on Tuesday morning, and one of your priority tasks is to pick up a prescription at the chemist on the high street, those tasks are bound by location. Your to-do list will also remind you to take the prescription with you when you're heading off for your appointment.

By task

Grouping tasks into one time block is extremely effective for saving you time. This idea applies to any task you do repeatedly. Grouping similar tasks into a time block and repeating that time block across a week, or even a month, creates a routine. This increases your productivity.

For example, if you're a blogger who needs to take photographs for upcoming posts, rather than taking a couple of photos every day, it's more productive to plan posts and images needed in advance, and take photos twice a month for a number of blog posts.

Or if one of your priority tasks is to make an important phone call, are there any other phone calls that might be less important but still need to be made? If you scheduled a certain amount of time, you could group all the phone calls together and get them all done. The important one would be completed first, then you'd make the other calls in your allocated time slot.

Scheduling specific times for phone calls and emails allows you to focus on more important work. It also means that you get through them more quickly; you can knock out one email or phone call after another, get them done and then move on. By the time you get to another block of 'phone and email time' later that day, or the next day, people will have had time to get back to you. *You take control* of when you reply.

Grouping together tasks related by activity or location makes you more efficient. Rather than jumping from task to task, you get all the same tasks done in one go or in one place. The more efficient you get at handling tasks, the quicker you'll get through your to-do list.

VISUAL CUES

In keeping with getting the list to work for you, you want to be able to see at a glance exactly what's done, what's in progress and what hasn't been started. You can use visual cues to help you see instantly how things stand.

Most people cross out tasks when they've been done; others tick them off or use a highlighter. This is fine – it shows what's done and what's not. However, many tasks can take a while to complete. Some tasks sit on our to-do list for days on end. We might be waiting for someone to return our email or call us back; we have to photocopy some documents or get to the post office.

Having loads of things still on the to-do list can be very overwhelming, which is why I find only having the pleasure of crossing something out at the very end a bit demotivating. You could be working your tail end off on a task and get no motivation from your list.

Most of the tasks on your list are in fact 'in progress'; you've started them but they're not finished yet. I like to indicate that on my list. It makes me feel better to know that even though some things aren't crossed off my list I'm still in control of them, and it shows me what I have started. What I do is tick (✓) tasks that are in progress; then, when the task is finished, I happily strike through the task and the tick.

Here's a list I used recently. Some tasks are ticked (in progress – started but not finished); some have a strike-through (complete); others have nothing next to them (not yet started).

DAILY TO-DO LIST WEDNESDAY 6 SEPTEMBER 2017	
HOME	WORK
✓ ~~Go food shopping~~	✓ ~~Attend breakfast meeting~~
Bring jeans for alteration	Look up images for book cover
Practise singing	✓ Prepare for client tomorrow
	✓ ~~Follow up on yesterday's emails~~
	3 x sales calls
	✓ ~~Buy office supplies~~

As you can see, I went to a meeting, got food shopping done, bought office supplies and followed up on yesterday's emails. All those tasks were started and fully completed. I started getting ready for the next day's client, but still had a bit more to do, so this item was ticked to indicate it was in progress.

By using these visual cues, I know what the status of each task is. Visual cues help our brain assess the situation at a glance, which in turn helps our productivity.

In addition, using a visual cue for tasks that are in progress gives me added motivation. I get the interim satisfaction of being able to place a mid-task tick rather than only getting that joy when a task is finished.

LET SOME TASKS GO

You probably won't be able to get through everything on your list, which is why prioritising is so important. If you run out of time and energy or get interrupted, at least you know you've got the most important tasks done.

If a task is continuously moved from week to week, however, you have two questions to answer. First, are you procrastinating? If so, this task needs to be of a higher priority for you. Second, do you *really* need to do this task? Could it be delegated to someone or perhaps eliminated completely? Make sure you don't hang on to to-dos because you are trying to be perfect and get everything done, or because you feel you 'should' hang on to them. Some to-dos never get done, so take the pressure off yourself, take them off the list and move on.

Lists can give you a lovely sense of accomplishment. You mightn't think you've got through much in your day, but a list will confirm that in fact you did! And then you get the added pleasure of crossing things off your list. You might even enjoy doing that so much that you'll add things you did to your list just so that you can cross them off! Or is that just me?

Organised people don't necessarily want to clear out their wardrobe or wash dishes in the evening. We'd all rather relax in front of the television. But we know that coming down to a tidy kitchen in the morning, or not struggling to find our work clothes, will mean less stress and an easier start to our day. We prioritise our upcoming time. We make time now to benefit us later.

As you work on your time management, logging your time needs to go alongside writing lists and completing tasks.

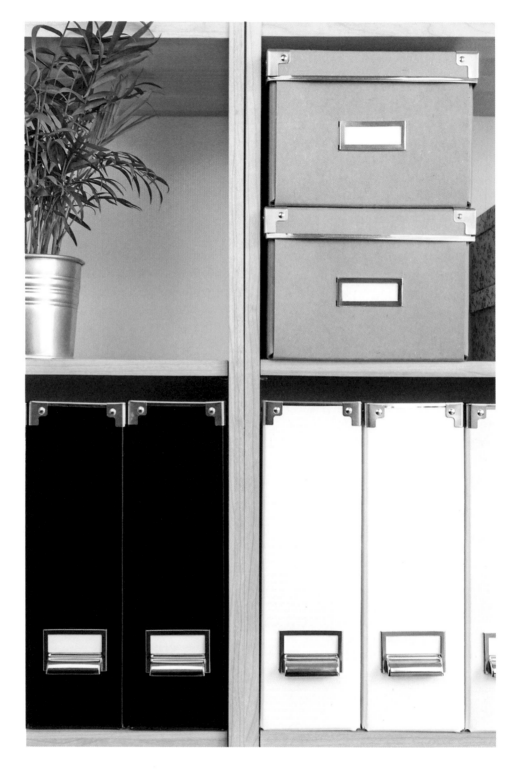

6

LOG IT

·

NOW YOU HAVE A
LIST A MILE LONG OF TO-DOS, BUT YOU'RE
STILL STUCK FOR TIME. LET THERE
BE NO PANIC!

·

In order to find time, you have to understand
where your time is going. Do you know how
long it takes you to do certain things?

·

For example, how long does it take you to:

- ✓ **MAKE YOUR BED**
- ✓ **COMMUTE TO AND FROM WORK**
- ✓ **MAKE SUNDAY DINNER**

And are there activities you never get time to do, such as exercising, reading, getting to bed early, going on a date with your partner, writing your novel …? If you guessed timings for the activities listed above, how many were accurate? If you feel that you never have enough time, there's a good chance your estimates aren't generous enough.

Getting control of your time is a work in progress. It involves doing a little experiment on yourself, then analysing what you find and putting a system in place. It takes motivation and discipline to create the system and follow it until it becomes a habit. Then you just 'know' how long things take and your estimates are much more accurate.

You can make changes to your time as follows:

1. **USING TIME LOGS**

2. **LAYING OUT WHAT YOU KNOW RIGHT NOW INTO A SCHEDULE**

3. **USING YOUR TIME LOGS TO IMPROVE THAT SCHEDULE**

Some people prefer not to draw up a schedule until they have assessed their time. If that is you, then you can stick with step one for the moment. Others want to put solutions in place immediately and then improve on them as they learn more through their time logs.

I personally think it's best to get started on a schedule (explained next) and then work on improving. Remember, you don't have to do everything perfectly. You just have to start.

Everyone can use time logs: stay-at-home parents, people in permanent and pensionable jobs, CEOs, bloggers, business owners working from home, entrepreneurs working remotely. Time logging simply means writing down everything you do and how long it takes you.

Here's an example of one of mine:

TIME LOG DATE: WEDNESDAY 28 JUNE		
TASK	TIME IT TOOK	NOTES
MEDITATION	10 mins	
COMMUTE	30 mins	
WALK	25 mins	
WORK/WRITING	4 hours	
COMMUTE	30 mins	
MAKING LUNCH	10 mins	
EATING LUNCH/RELAXING	45 mins	
SALES CALLS	30 mins	
ANSWERING EMAILS	15 mins	

Time logs are useful because we usually grossly underestimate how long things take. We underestimate for various reasons, for example: we don't break the tasks down enough; we think we have enough time to add in 'one more thing'; and we don't add any contingency time.

As a result, we run late. We don't get everything done we wanted or needed to. Or somehow we do manage to arrive on time and get everything done but we're exhausted and stressed because of the time pressure and effort.

So we're back to how tasks are broken down and why. Everything you need to do should have a 'when' you will do it next to it. You can't assign the appropriate day and time to a task if you can't estimate how long it will take. Assigning time well means laying out an effective schedule for yourself. This means that you need to make a breakdown of each task and log an approximate time for each part of the task.

One of our earlier examples was 'Organise Oliver's birthday party'. If all you need to do is note the date of that event, then putting 'Organise Oliver's birthday party' in your calendar is enough.

However, if organising the party involves multiple sub-tasks, just writing 'Organise Oliver's birthday party' on your to-do list is going to lead you into major time trouble. Effective time management involves detailing every single task associated with that event and assigning each task to a specific time.

As we saw before, birthday organisation involves these steps:

- ✓ **ORDER BIRTHDAY CAKE**
- ✓ **COLLECT BIRTHDAY CAKE**
- ✓ **BUY CANDLES**
- ✓ **BUY GIFT AND CARD**
- ✓ **BUY DECORATIONS**
- ✓ **CREATE INVITATIONS**
- ✓ **POST/DELIVER INVITATIONS**
- ✓ **CONFIRM ATTENDEES**
- ✓ **CLEAN THE HOUSE**

Ordering the birthday cake is going to involve a phone call. Are there other phone calls you can make at the same time (remember grouping tasks together)? Yes? How long will the phone calls take now?

You need to collect the birthday cake. Can you do that when you go food shopping? Can you get someone else to collect it?

You need to buy a gift and card. Have you a stash of cards already in the house? Yes? How long will it take to find them? Can you get the gift locally or does it involve online shopping? If so, you will need to be aware of delivery dates.

See how much time everything takes?

The more you log time and plan ahead, the more you get used to it. It might seem like a lot of questions and a lot of work, but some people do it all in their head very quickly because they're used to it. You will be too, if you put the practice in.

We have tasks that we need to do on our Daily to-do list. Then we have tasks we do naturally during the course of the day that might not be on a list but need to be assessed time-wise too, such as driving to the shops for the groceries or taking an evening shower.

By understanding your time, you will understand your schedule. By understanding your schedule, you can prioritise. You can cut things out at short notice if you need. You can assign extra time to other tasks should that be necessary.

If you are constantly chasing time and trying to catch up, you don't have that luxury.

OVER TO YOU!

In order to assess your time, create your own Time Log, as in the example above. Photocopy seven of them and track where your time goes over the next week. If you can stretch to two weeks, all the better. Write down everything you do and the time it took. By the end of that week or fortnight, you will see patterns:

- Tasks that are repeated
- Whether those tasks are repeated on the same days or at similar times of day
- The average time those repetitive tasks take
- Whether tasks that *could* be done together *are* being done together
- If there are tasks that take too long

- If there are tasks that cause pressure and need extra time

- If there are tasks that you could drop (when the effort or time taken is greater than the return for doing them)

- If there are tasks that can be delegated to others

Stop double-jobbing

Unconsciously, we prolong a task when there is no need. When you find items that don't belong in the room you are organising, don't go back and forth distributing them to where they should go. If you zig-zag back and forth, you will make the whole decluttering process much longer than it needs to be. You're also more likely to get distracted by things to do in the other rooms. Stay where you are!

Or you leave mis-matched items out in your eye-line until you find its mate instead of simply putting it away or throwing it out and doing the same with the match when it's found. Or you find yourself up and down from the printer all afternoon instead of lining up all required documents and printing in one go.

Don't make things harder on yourself!

Also, don't confuse grouping tasks as we discussed in the previous chapter with multitasking. By grouping tasks you are doing similar work over an extended period of time or in the same location. Multi-tasking is doing two or more different tasks at the same time. You can do neither job efficiently as a result. Double-jobbing involves multiple attempts at what is effectively the same task. It all results in mistakes, time wasting, delays and lower productivity.

Two minutes or less

The work you are doing now is the most important thing, but sometimes something unexpected will come up. Use the two-minute idea to determine if you should deal with it now or assign time for it later on. If you can do it in two minutes or less, do so. You have to be very disciplined for this, so beware. If it takes longer than two minutes, leads on to other tasks or results in daydreaming, leave it until later.

Just one more thing

Don't be the 'just one more thing' person. Imagine you have to be somewhere at 11 o'clock and it takes you 30 minutes to get there. You are ready to leave at 10.20. Instead of leaving now and taking your time getting there, you think, 'I'll just put the bins out.' This either makes you late, or puts you under pressure to make your appointment.

We all do it: we think we've just got time to water the plants, make a quick phone call or feed the cats. Sometimes it works out, but often it leads to delays, accidents and stress. Having a little window of time is good. Don't ruin it by adding one more thing.

Contingency

Even better than a small window of extra time is assigning contingency time to your schedule. Contingency time is your lifeline. At the start, when you're getting used to this new way of managing time and re-evaluating the time you have, always err on the side of caution. Better to over-estimate and have a few extra minutes to do something or arrive a few minutes early than to be always up against it.

I usually add an extra 15 minutes to anything I'm doing. Even if I'm running late, if I've got a 15-minute buffer I should arrive just on time.

For large projects, estimating the time it will take to complete the project and then doubling it gives you leeway. Adding in contingency time is a good habit to develop.

Time logging takes practice. As you try it out, you will almost certainly over-extend yourself again and learn more about the time tasks really take and the space you need for them in your schedule.

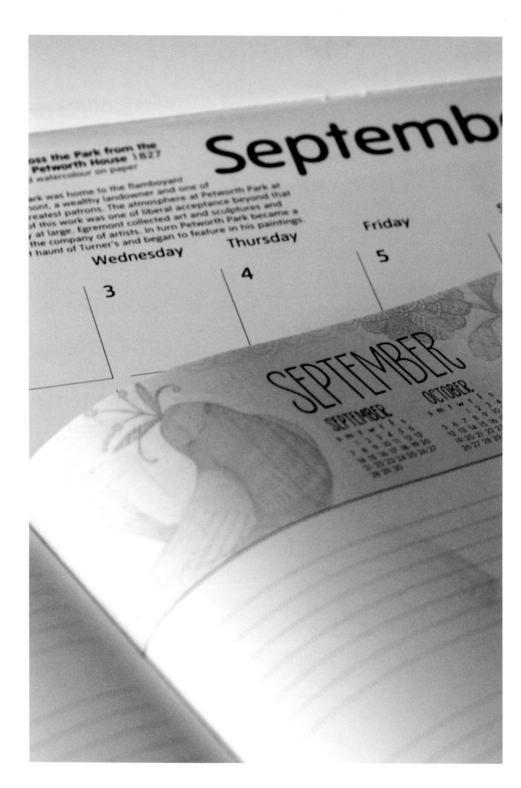

...oss the Park from the
...Petworth House 1827
...watercolour on paper

...rk was home to the flamboyant
...ont, a wealthy landowner and one of
...reatest patrons. The atmosphere at Petworth Park at
...of this work was one of liberal acceptance beyond that
...y at large. Egremont collected art and sculptures and
...the company of artists. In turn Petworth Park became a
...haunt of Turner's and began to feature in his paintings.

September

Wednesday	Thursday	Friday
3	4	5

SEPTEMBER

7

LAY IT OUT

·

AS BUSY ADULTS, WE NEED TO HAVE AN IDEA OF OUR TIME AND YET WE OFTEN DON'T THINK ABOUT IT AS A STRUCTURED FORMAT.

·

When you were in school, every day was clearly laid out in your school timetable. Even after-school activities, such as sports practice or homework clubs, were factored in. Schedules are an adult's school timetable.

·

Don't confuse your schedule with your calendar. Calendars are for keeping track of appointments, birthdays, events that are coming up. While these are also noted on a schedule, most calendars don't allow more in-depth tracking.

Schedules break down your day into minute detail. Calendars don't generally have this facility: online calendars that do allow you to break down your day into units are really schedules rather than calendars. While a calendar can note the deadline for a certain goal, it doesn't factor in the actionable steps to get there that a schedule facilitates.

BREAKING DOWN YOUR DAY

When you are creating or choosing your schedule you need to decide two things:

1   DO YOU WANT A MONDAY–FRIDAY SCHEDULE OR A SEVEN-DAY SCHEDULE?

2   DO YOU WANT TO BREAK THE DAY DOWN BY HOUR OR ON THE HALF HOUR?

On page 70-71 you'll see an example of a seven-day schedule broken down by hour. You can use this sample to create your own.

YOUR ENERGY CYCLE

Before you start to lay out your schedule, think about your energy cycle.

Whether you're a morning person or a night owl, it's very important to assign your most difficult and most important tasks to the time of day when you feel most energetic. Leave tasks lower down the priority scale for times of the day when you are less energetic. I'm hopeless in the afternoon, for example, so I schedule easy tasks then.

If you're a morning person and need to organise the spare room, do it first thing. You'll get more done if you schedule it for the morning. Then, as your energy lags in the afternoon, sit down and call the insurance broker or book your car service. Or, if you work best in the evening, schedule writing your thesis after dinner.

FILLING UP YOUR SCHEDULE

There are many moving parts to a good schedule. Once you have decided which type you will use, start filling in the schedule.

I **START WITH THE ACTIVITIES YOU KNOW ABOUT ALREADY.** Some of them will be the same every week. For example: the time you get to work and leave work; when you need to collect children from school; the kids' after-school activities that you need to bring them to and/or attend; any appointments for the week; any classes you take; any arrangements you have made with friends.

2 **NEXT, PUT IN PRIORITIES THAT YOU JUST CAN'T MOVE.** Check your diary or your phone and/or with your partner and make sure you don't forget anything.

3 **NOW ADD ITEMS THAT YOU MIGHT NEVER HAVE CONSIDERED PUTTING INTO A SCHEDULE.** For example, you know you need to have dinner, but have you put it into the schedule? What about the time required to make it, eat it and clear up? You know you'll be having a shower, but would you have scheduled it into your day before now? In it goes to your new schedule.

Steps one, two and three here are more effectively scheduled the more information you get from your time log. Have a look at the sample schedule that I have filled in by completing steps one, two and three. Pockets of available time are clearly visible. These are filled up by completing step four – adding in the Daily to-do list.

4 **ADD YOUR DAILY TO-DO LIST.** Once you've finished steps 1–3, look at your schedule and identify where your pockets of time are, if any. It's these pockets of time that you will use to start clearing the tasks on your Daily to-do list.

For every to-do you write down, you need to write down *when* you are going to do it. Think of your to-do list as a When To Do List.

By now you have created a to-do list for the week and you have chosen your priority tasks. It's time to schedule those tasks into your week. The first task to schedule is your number one priority task. Get the number one task done first, out of the way, and move on with your day. Aim to get at least five top tasks into your schedule over the week – one per weekday.

FACTORING IN YOUR TIME LOG

Schedules can be created from today to help you manage your time better. They can be in use as you start logging time for the various tasks that you do. As the time logs start to build up and show you a story of how long tasks take, you can use this information to improve your schedules.

Start your schedule with your best estimate of time. As you get more experienced in estimating time, you can assign bigger or smaller time blocks in your schedule. Don't forget your contingency time – this needs to be reflected in your schedule too.

IN ORDER TO GET ORGANISED, YOU NEED TO GET AHEAD OF THE CLUTTER.

	MONDAY	TUESDAY	WEDNESDAY
	WEEKLY SCHEDULE BY HOUR		
06.00-07.00			
07.00-08.00			
08.00-09.00	Commute/kids to school	Commute/kids to school	Commute/kids to school
09.00-10.00	Work	Work	Work
10.00-11.00	Work	Work	Work
11.00-12.00	Work	Work	Work
12.00-13.00	Work	Work	Work
13.00-14.00	Lunch	Lunch	Lunch/Food shopping
14.00-15.00	Work	Work	Work
15.00-16.00	Work	Work	Work
16.00-17.00	Work	Work	Work
17.00-18.00	Commute/Collect kids	Commute/Collect kids	Commute/Collect kids
18.00-19.00	Dinner	Dinner/drive to Pilates	Dinner
19.00-20.00		Pilates class	
20.00-21.00	Kids' bedtime routine	Drive home/ shower	Kids' bedtime routine
21.00-22.00	Kids' bedtime routine/ TV	Kids' bedtime routine/ TV	Kids' bedtime routine/ TV
22.00-23.00	Prep tomorrow/Bedtime	Prep tomorrow/Bedtime	Prep tomorrow/Bedtime

THURSDAY	FRIDAY	SATURDAY	SUNDAY
Drive to dentist	Commute/kids to school		Drive to rugby
Family Dental appt.	Work		Kids Rugby
Commute to work/ school	Work	Drive to hair appt.	Kids Rugby
Work	Work	Hair Appt.	Kids Rugby
Work	Work	Food Shopping	Drive home
Lunch	Lunch/Go to bank	Drive home/ Unpack shopping	Lunch
Work	Work		
Work	Work		
Work	Work		Drive to parents
Commute/Collect kids	Commute/Collect kids		Visit parents
Dinner	Dinner		Visit parents
		Night out	Return home
Kids' bedtime routine	Kids' bedtime routine	Night out	
Kids' bedtime routine/ TV	Kids' bedtime routine/ TV	Night out	
Prep tomorrow/Bedtime	Prep tomorrow/Bedtime	Night out	

You should now see pockets of time emerging that you can use for your declutter and organisation projects. Alternatively, there may be unavailable blocks of time that are filled with activities that are less important and less urgent and could be swapped for decluttering and organising, if you so wish.

In order to get organised, you need to get ahead of the clutter. Stuff comes into our lives on an everyday basis. Some people only declutter once every six months; others stop after decluttering and don't think through how they use their space. As a result, there is never any real organisational transformation.

However, if you sort out blocks of time and make a commitment to work consistently on organisation, you will make a greater impact. Initially the blocks of time needed for decluttering and organising will have to be significant in length, for example, taking three days off work, or blocking out every morning for two weeks.

However, as you reduce what you own and put some organisation on what is staying, you'll need shorter blocks of time. Finally, you'll move into maintenance mode, when you'll only need 15 minutes at the end of the day to tidy up, or you'll spend Sunday evenings scheduling your week or assign Saturday mornings to cleaning the home. At this stage, you can afford to declutter only every six months because the home runs itself. Aside from the regular mess expected from a busy household, it's now a mere cleaning issue rather than a huge clutter situation.

But to get to that point, you need to call time out on running around the hamster wheel gathering clutter with each rotation. *Step out, analyse, reassess* and build a new system that works. This is done through time.

Once you have added in times for your organisation projects, you have now completed your weekly schedule and it's ready to be consulted and used for the week. You can now see how your week is going to run in one snapshot. If there are any last-minute changes, interruptions or emergencies, you can clearly see what you can either drop completely or move to another day or another week to accommodate this change of circumstance.

This schedule is a system in your external environment that helps you keep track of everything you need to do and when and where you need to be.

When you have it written down, all this information is no longer flying around your brain. You're not struggling to sleep with everything you have to do running through your head. You don't wake up at three in the morning in a panic over something you've forgotten. You don't forget important dates and can plan for events ahead of time. It eases the burden on your brain and offers you a chance to get to things in an orderly, organised and timely manner, without stress.

We live in a very fast-paced world. We can't control the circumstances and situations around us. We can only control our responses to them. If we're under too much pressure, something has to give and usually it's our health or our relationships. How far are you going to push these two aspects of your life before you realise something has to change?

Our family, kids, colleagues, bosses, the economic situation – all put pressure on our time. Every day what they do influences us. But it's up to us what we do with this information – how we interpret it, react to it and ultimately manage it.

Ironically, if we want things to slow down, we have to take time out in order to reassess and strategise, none of which is easy. But all of which is up to us.

Understanding your time, your priorities and your goals makes you clearer on what you say 'yes' and 'no' to. Once you have identified the time available to declutter and have scheduled to do so, it's time to get stuck into organising your space.

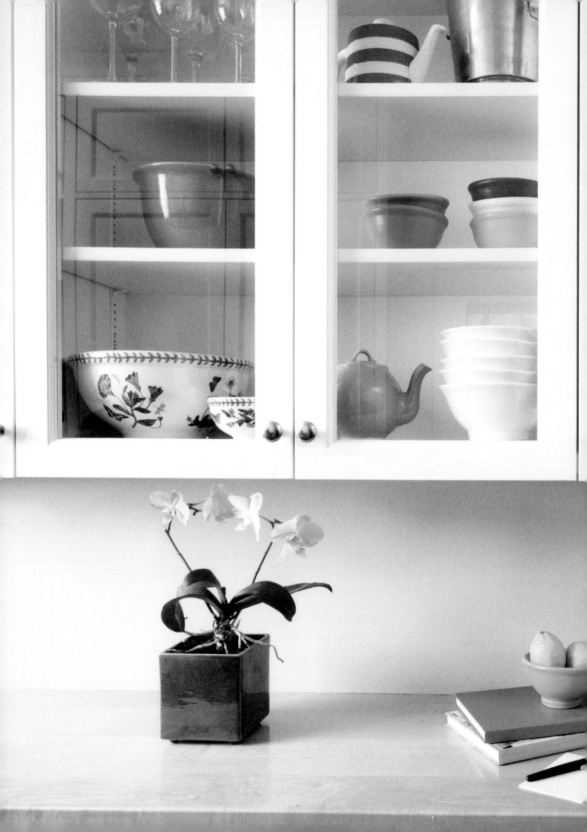

Part III

Your Space

·

'IT ALWAYS SEEMS
IMPOSSIBLE UNTIL IT'S DONE.'

NELSON MANDELA

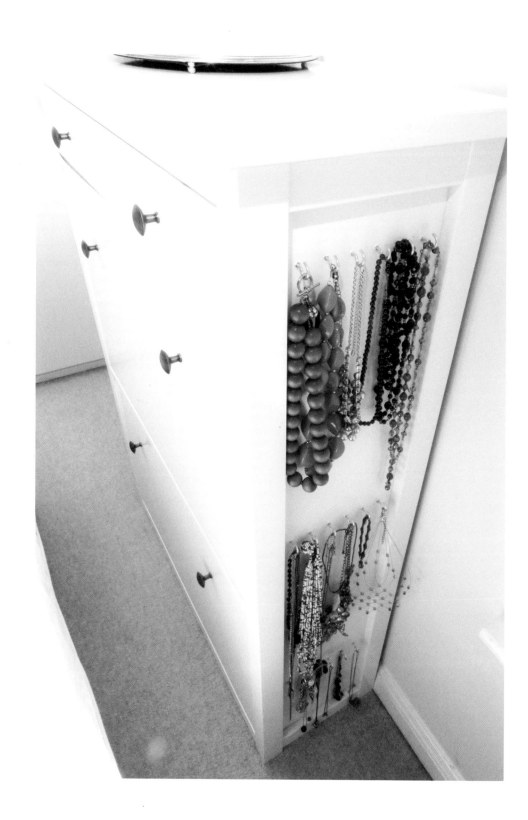

8

THE METHOD

•

WHEN WAS THE LAST TIME YOU TOOK A WALK AROUND YOUR HOME AND JUST OBSERVED?

•

Probably never, right? You bought (or rented) it, moved in, had plans – some of which you did, others you said you'd get back to. And since then, more stuff has been bought, some decor changed, perhaps a child or two added to the mix or maybe just a cat. Life goes on and yet you feel the house clutter is increasing and it doesn't look as you imagined it would. Time to take a step back and take an aerial view of things.

•

Take a pen and paper or your phone and walk from room to room. Take note of the following:

- WHAT DIY NEEDS TO BE DONE (INCLUDING ANY EASY PAINTING JOBS)?

- WHAT LARGE PIECES OF FURNITURE COULD GO? (TO SELL, DONATE, GIVE TO FRIENDS/FAMILY, MOVE TO THE ATTIC)

- ARE THERE ANY OTHER ITEMS YOU ARE CONSIDERING SELLING?

- WHAT LARGE PIECES OF FURNITURE ACTUALLY BELONG IN A DIFFERENT ROOM?

- ARE THERE ANY ITEMS THAT BELONG TO OTHER PEOPLE AND NEED TO BE RETURNED?

- WHAT ITEMS HAVE YOU ALREADY DECIDED TO DONATE BUT HAVEN'T DONE SO YET?

- WHAT ITEMS COULD EASILY BE ADDED TO THE DONATION PILE?

- IS THERE ARTWORK TO BE HUNG UP, OR PHOTOGRAPHS TO BE FRAMED AND/OR HUNG UP?

- WHAT HEAVY ITEMS WOULD YOU LIKE TO MOVE IF YOU HAD SOME HELP?

Don't do any tidying of any kind. Don't bring items from one room to another. This is purely an observation and note-taking exercise. The aim is to help you see the story your house is telling you.

At the end of this walk around you should have a few lists to hand, such as:

- DIY TO BE DONE

- ITEMS TO BE SOLD

- ITEMS TO BE RETURNED TO OTHER PEOPLE

- DONATIONS

Some of the clutter and disorganisation in our homes often comes from unfinished jobs. Simply rectifying some of those odd jobs can make a difference to your space.

For example, you'll notice I put 'easy painting jobs' on the list above. Big painting and decorating jobs are projects and belong on a separate list. Only small irritations and unfinished jobs that are quick to turn around should go on this list: pictures that need to be hung; kitchen cabinet or wardrobe doors that are hanging off the hinges; wonky drawers; blinds that need adjusting, etc.

When things aren't working properly we can't use them properly. If we can't use them, they and the items that are affected by their not working become clutter. They also become a to-do for us.

Many of these minor jobs can be done by one good handyman or handywoman. Hire someone for one day, hand them the list and by dinner time all those irritating to-dos will be done and dusted! And all you had to do was write a list and make a booking. Easy, isn't it? No drama.

AVOID GRAND DESIGNS

At this point, we are not looking at big renovation or interior design plans.

Many people who call me think that all they need are some storage ideas. Others have grand designs and plans that they're considering in order to create more space. They're not wrong – an extension or storage may work very well – but that's not where to start. Clients often talk about their plans for a kitchen extension, or a new laundry room, or knocking one side of the house to extend the size of the downstairs. They are fantastic, exciting goals to have, but they take a lot of time, effort and money. And what do you have to do first before any of that? Declutter.

You're probably already surrounded by clutter, or you feel that nothing has a proper home. You're feeling overwhelmed by it and by lack of time. If you're working full time, and if you have young children, there's an awful lot going on. And now you're going to add an extension and all the stress that comes with it? But at least when it's finished you'll feel more in control, right? Well, let's take a breath for a moment. Let's just plan this out from where you are to where you want to be. An extension is another item to buy. More rooms and more storage do not necessarily mean more space – either physically or mentally and certainly not financially.

Let's start with the existing space first. There are ways of getting this space working better before you do anything else. And there are several reasons why you should do this, whether or not you end up going for that extension or renovation. Right now, the reason for the renovation is 'I need more space'. But why? *Why* do you need more space? How will you use the space? What will you fill the space with?

By decluttering and going through the space you already have and the items you own, you will be able to examine in close detail how you are using the space you currently have. Once you have reduced what you own and organised the space, you can identify exactly what is going on in the home, what family habits are not working in the space. As a result, you can construct – literally – a solution. You can present an inventory to architects and interior designers and clearly state not only where you lack space but why.

✓ **WHAT HAPPENS IF YOU BUILD A WARDROBE AND IT ONLY HAS SIX DRAWERS?** It looked gorgeous in the brochure and the plans were exciting. But now, as you fill the wardrobe, you realise that six drawers only hold underwear for you and your partner. What about T-shirts? Pyjamas? Sportswear? You'll have to hang those up now.

✓ **IF YOU HAD ARRANGED THE OLD WARDROBE SPACE WITH THE ITEMS YOU ALREADY OWN**, you could have identified clearly what worked and what didn't. You could have assessed what items you wanted folded, what items would be better hung up, etc.

✓ **AND WHAT ABOUT YOUR SHOES?** Shoes are one of the biggest problem in people's homes nowadays. I have yet to find a wardrobe that facilitates storing shoes. It's as if they're an afterthought. Kids grow out of shoes so quickly that it's normal to find several different sizes of shoes. They are also handed from one child to the next, so one pair could do the rounds for years. There are also many different types of shoe – sports shoes, hiking boots, Wellington boots, ski boots, rollerblades. No one thinks of them until they notice that they have been hanging around in the hall all year.

✓ **SO YOU DESIGN YOUR WARDROBE, A SECTION OF YOUR UTILITY ROOM OR UNDER THE STAIRS TO CATER FOR SHOES.** But do you know how many shoes are actually going to fit in the storage provided? For instance, pull-out rails in wardrobes look great, but they hold four pairs maximum. So how many will you need?

✓ **WHEN YOU ORGANISE YOUR EXISTING WARDROBE AND NEATLY ARRANGE YOUR SHOES IN THE SPACE, CHANCES ARE THEY'RE NOT ALL GOING TO FIT.** Which is why you want a new wardrobe. In that instance, you line up all the shoes that don't fit and take note of it for your new design. Now you know exactly how many pairs of shoes need a home. You can then tell your wardrobe designer exactly what you need. You couldn't do that if you hadn't decluttered and organised your existing space first. Telling a designer, 'I want ten shelves holding eight pairs of shoes,' is much better than 'I need space for shoes.'

Going in head first and hoping for the best is what got you into the situation you are currently in. You end up forcing your stuff into a new space, instead of your space fitting what you own. Spatial design is one thing, but an inventory in conjunction with your space is essential. Otherwise you're just hedging your bets.

By all means, make plans for your grand designs, but one way or another, decluttering is going to be part of your plans, and it would save time and money to *declutter wisely first*.

ORGANISING SESSIONS

Decluttering flows from one room to another. The kitchen will flow into the utility room, which may flow into your hallway or under the stairs. The bedroom wardrobe may flow into the spare room wardrobe, which will flow into the spare room itself and then perhaps the attic.

Getting ahead of the clutter is key. The way to do that is to declutter in regular blocks of time, which is why we looked at your time in Part II. If you're going to declutter, declutter efficiently. There's no point sorting through your wardrobe on Saturday, then leaving it for a few weeks and coming back to sort out the rest of the bedroom three weeks later. Like following a fitness plan, once you decide to do it, you need to do it regularly. Regular sessions in quick succession will get you a result and get it over with a lot more quickly than dragging it out over a long period.

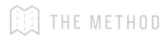 ## THE METHOD

In Part II we looked at 'completing the circle' and breaking down tasks into Preparation → Task → Clear-up. Now, your task is decluttering and there will be work to do beforehand and afterwards so that you get the job done and the result you want. Whether you tackle a small bathroom cupboard or a large garage, the method before, during and after is the same.

PREPARATION

No matter what you decide to organise – paper, a wardrobe, kitchen cupboards, cables, photos – you need to prepare first. Preparation is broken into three parts:

1 GATHER YOUR ORGANISING TOOLS

2 SET A TIME LIMIT

3 TIDY UP

GATHER YOUR ORGANISING TOOLS

When you're cooking, you line up your ingredients before you start. In the same way, you can't organise without some aids. Think of what you will need to get the work done and get them prepared first before you start anything. It will only take five minutes to grab the things you need, but it will save you a lot of time, effort and frustration.

For every organising session, you will need:

✓ LARGE CLEAR SPACE TO SPREAD OUT AND WORK ON

✓ BLACK MARKER

✓ POST-IT NOTES/BLANK PAPER

✓ POLISH, CLOTHS, WIPES

✓ MUSIC/RADIO (IF THAT HELPS YOU)

✓ CUP OF TEA/COFFEE/WATER

✓ CLOCK/WATCH/TIMER

For paperwork, you might need to add the following:

✓ LABELS

✓ PAPERCLIPS

✓ STAPLER

✓ YOUR FILING SYSTEM – LEVER-ARCH FOLDERS/DROP-DOWN FILES/
FILING CABINET

✓ SHREDDER

For a wardrobe, you might need to add:

✓ SELECTION OF HANGERS

✓ IRON AND IRONING BOARD

No matter what area you're organising, you'll also need at least four bags/bins/
boxes, labelled:

✓ GENERAL RUBBISH/RECYCLING

✓ CHARITY DONATIONS

✓ TO BE RETURNED (E.G. LIBRARY BOOKS, A DISH BELONGING TO
YOUR MOTHER)

✓ BELONGS ELSEWHERE IN THE HOME

If you're prepared in advance, and have everything to hand, you can focus and
get down to the job without getting distracted.

SET A TIME LIMIT

One of the biggest challenges in organising space is the overwhelming feeling that comes with doing this work. It can be a big task. Every fibre of your being wishes you were doing anything but this.

To create and maintain focus, a time limit will help. Be organised in your thinking. *Be realistic.* Look at the space you're about to tackle. Is it a small bathroom cabinet, a junk drawer, or a garage? Have a realistic expectation of what you will get done and the time you have available to do it.

Block out your time. Instead of saying 'I'll work on this for the morning', be specific. Give it an exact time, for example 'two hours', 'from 9 a.m. to 11 a.m.' or 'from 9 a.m. to 10 a.m., then I'll have a ten-minute coffee break and go again from 10.10 a.m. to 11.30 a.m.'.

TIDY UP

Organising can be a messy affair! I often tell my clients that the place might get worse before it gets better. They are already swamped in clutter, so this isn't really what they want to hear. The reality is that you are, after all, about to pull out a load of things you've avoided looking at for God knows how long, so this in itself will create a mess. You'll also be finding things a new home, so it's going to involve moving things around a bit.

In order to reduce the mess, I always encourage people to do a surface clean before starting any organising. When an area is generally clean it is easier to organise the area. There are several reasons for this. When the 'organising mess' starts to emerge, you are not putting one mess on top of another. You know that the mess you are looking at is purely the stuff you are trying to organise. So once you get through this, the room will be back to its clean state.

Putting one mess on top of another causes stress and frustration. You will think the situation is worse than it actually is, you'll start thinking, 'Oh God, I can't keep organising this, look at the mess I'll have to clear up,' and you'll stop. Unless you clean up a bit beforehand, most of the mess you're looking at now was already there before you even started.

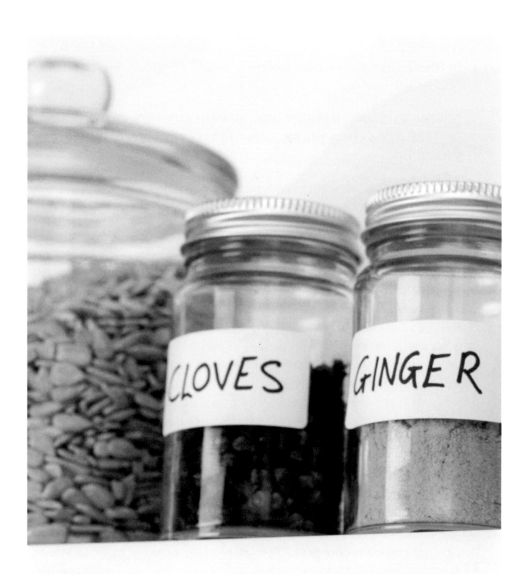

Organising is what I call a 'deep clean', and it's much easier to do if you first do a 'surface clean' – a quick general clear-up of the space.

- ✓ IN THE KITCHEN, CLEAN THE COUNTERS, WASH THE DISHES, BRUSH THE FLOOR.

- ✓ FOR THE WARDROBE, MAKE THE BED, OPEN THE CURTAINS, PUT AWAY ANY CLOTHES (YES, EVEN IF YOU ARE GOING TO TAKE THEM OUT AGAIN IN A MINUTE!)

- ✓ IN THE BEDROOM, PICK EVERYTHING UP OFF THE FLOOR AND PUT IT ALL ON YOUR BED. HAVING THE FLOOR CLEARED INSTANTLY MAKES THE ROOM LOOK BETTER AND YOU CAN MOVE AROUND MORE EASILY.

In some rooms, such as laundry rooms, toy rooms or spare rooms, you may be thinking that you can't tidy up because there's no space. You may need to take large items out of the room. If you do move items outside, keep them close, such as in an adjacent hallway or room, and make sure that the hallway or other room is tidy before you do so. For example, if your hall is a bit messy already and then you add clutter from the spare room, it will drive you nuts. So tidy the hallway and then create space in your spare room to work. Be very selective with what you move out. Keep it to a minimum because you really need to look at as much as possible in this room in one go.

When we organise, we pull everything out, leaving us with a clean slate; a blank canvas that we can rebuild in a better way. Every item we pull out will be categorised, so you will need somewhere to spread all these items out. If you're tackling the kitchen, for example, make sure that your kitchen table and/or kitchen island are clean and clear. If you're sorting out the garden shed, place a rug outside on the grass. If you're working on a toy room and there's no flat surface, maybe clear the kitchen table so that you can work from there.

Always start your organising session with a clean room and a clear, flat surface to help you keep items together and prevent other items getting mixed up in your new organised system.

Now we'll move on to the task of decluttering the space we are in. This task is broken into three parts:

1   CATEGORISE

2   DECLUTTER

3   ORGANISE

From a bedside locker to an attic, you start by creating categories for every item in the space. Once that is done, taking one category at a time, you declutter. Remove items you no longer need, love or use, and put them in the bin, for recycling or ready for donation. Once you know what you're keeping, you compare the available space you have with each category of items.

Organising involves examining the furniture and storage you already have and the space it gives you and comparing or matching it up with the sizes of the different categories you have created. Some items will go back where they came from; for other items, you create new homes. When new homes are created, sometimes storage is needed.

Often people don't organise until they have the right storage, but you should always buy storage *after* decluttering. Once we know what we want to keep and where we are going to put things, we can make better choices for our storage. You can always 'home' items while waiting on the purchase of storage. For example, if you have more books than you have shelving, place the books you can on your current bookcase and then line up the reminder of the books next to it. The amount of space these spare books take up now highlights the size of bookcase you need. But the books themselves can sit neatly to the side until you get to buy one. You can still organise the books and give them a home. Storage will be added later to finalise the organisation.

So how exactly do you categorise, declutter and organise?

CATEGORISE

Organising in its simplest form is separating things into categories – putting like with like. The first step is to separate your things into categories. Put together things that are related or that belong together. No more finding your shampoo next to the cat food. Categorising is something we do automatically anyway, whether or not we're aware of it.

CREATING CATEGORIES

You need to see exactly what you are dealing with. Doing that involves pulling everything out and having a look. If it's a cardboard box full of miscellaneous items, toss it all upside down out onto the large area where you are working. If it's a shelf or a cabinet or a drawer, take everything out. You need to see everything; you need to know exactly what you own.

Remember, in our preparation stage we cleared the bed, the kitchen table or a section of floor so we could spread everything out. When you are categorising, imagine the flat surface as a grid of imaginary squares. Every category you create will be placed inside a square. This will keep your work neat and methodical. You can easily keep track of the categories and be organised from the very beginning.

Every time you pick up an item you will follow this process.

✓ LOOK AT THE FIRST ITEM. WHAT IS IT? WHAT'S THE FIRST WORD THAT COMES TO MIND? DON'T OVER-THINK IT. WHATEVER DESCRIPTION COMES TO MIND WHEN YOU LOOK AT THE ITEM, USE THAT. YOU ARE MORE LIKELY TO THINK OF THAT WORD NEXT TIME YOU NEED TO LOCATE THE ITEM.

✓ WRITE THE WORD ON A POST-IT OR PIECE OF PAPER AND PLACE IT NEXT TO THE ITEM.

✓ REPEAT THE PROCESS WITH THE NEXT ITEM.

✓ CATEGORIES WILL EMERGE AS YOU CONTINUE. WITH EACH ITEM, YOU WILL EITHER CREATE A NEW CATEGORY OR ADD IT TO A CATEGORY YOU HAVE ALREADY CREATED.

For example, take a selection of pens, crayons and pencils. Some people will identify all items as 'pens'; someone else might call it 'stationery' and add a stapler, scissors and paperclips into the category; someone else might name this group 'arts and crafts'; someone else will name it 'school supplies'. Or you might categorise all baking trays, tins and equipment as 'baking', but someone else might split the items into 'everyday baking' and 'kids' baking'.

Categories don't have to be made up of one or two words. Some of the most efficient categories take a sentence to explain. For example, if we're organising stationery, you could categorise some of it as 'Items I need to write my thesis'.

Or on a large scale, when I organise a particularly messy room, it may take a few days to get through it all, so I will organise what I can with the client over a few hours and push everything still to do to the other side of the room. I am categorising the room: on one side is what is done and the other side is categorised as 'still to do', or 'to be done at the next session'.

Often, there are times when individual items that have nothing to do with each other are brought together into a category. For example, a passport, wallet, toiletries, bottle of water and snack have nothing to do with each other, but they could all fit into the category 'things I need when travelling'.

To make it easier on yourself, pull out the easy items first – the things you immediately know how to categorise. This way you'll quickly reduce the amount of things you need to go through; you'll feel better about getting off to a good start; and you'll begin getting into the habit of grouping things together.

If you get stuck on an item – you're not sure what it is, how you would use it, when you might need it or where you would put it – just leave it to one side and keep going with the other items. As other categories emerge you may find a place for it. You may even find that when you come back to it a second time you decide to let it go. This happens 90 per cent of the time with my clients. The point is not to dwell. Keep going – you've enough to be getting on with!

Categories can take a while to emerge, so don't get disheartened if you find it tough going. At first, you may feel as though you are creating loads of categories with only one item in each group. This is often the case when you are dealing with paperwork. However, as you keep going, some categories will have more in them than others and your dominant groups will emerge.

There's no right or wrong way to categorise. The way you categorise something may not be the way I do it, and vice versa. Organising can be as individual as people. There are different ways to do it. How you categorise is down to you and what makes sense for you, how you use your space and your habits.

Now we're really getting to the nitty gritty of organising. When you're starting off, stick to one broad category. It's easier, quicker and will give you a good level of organisation. This is one-tier organisation.

However, the more organised you want to be, the more you need to get to grips with sub-categories. We tend to sub-divide if we have a lot of items in one broad category. A three-tier sub-division is the furthest I would ever go. It gets far too complicated after that and there's a danger of over-categorising. Here are two examples of categorising and sub-categorising what you own. Remember, there are many ways to categorise and how you do it is up to you!

For example, in a toy room, you might have very broad categories such as toys, books, technology, games. There are loads of different types of toys, pieces of technology, books and games in each category but you're not worried about further organisation. This is one-tier organisation.

However, if you do want to organise further, you could sub-divide the toys, for example, and break them down more specifically by type (two-tier).

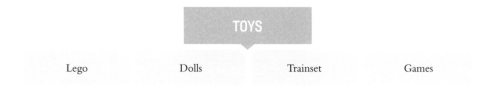

Or you could divide them up by child and then by type (three-tier).

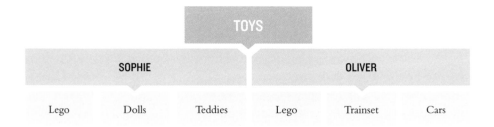

Similarly, in a bedroom, you may have broad categories such as clothes, jewellery, books, shoes, bedlinen. There are different types of clothes, jewellery etc. in each category, but you're happy keeping it simple. That's one-tiered organisation.

If you wanted to be more specific, you could sub-categorise clothes, for instance. You could divide by type (two-tier). Or, just like the toys, you could divide by person and then by type (three-tier).

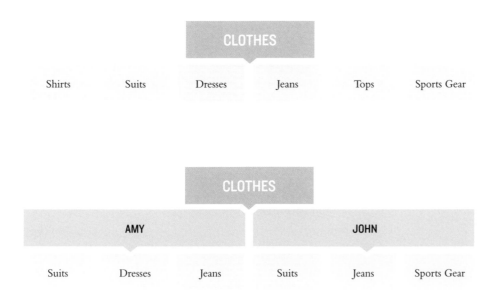

CATEGORISATION BY COLOUR CODING

If you decide to colour code your categories, you have graduated from organising school! This is the ultimate in organisation.

Colour coding the wardrobe

We've often heard advice to colour code clothes on the wardrobe rail to keep them organised. For some people it works and it looks amazing, especially if you add matching hangers. However, I often find it hard to differentiate clothes if I've grouped them by colour. Particularly black clothes – I have a lot of black! The whole point of getting organised and organising your things is to make life simpler, not harder. So if I want a black shirt, and I'm wading through every other black article, it's causing a delay and the system isn't working. But colour coding your clothes is certainly worth trying out, if you think it will work for you. You can always try it and if it doesn't work you can try something that suits you better.

One alternative is to colour code your hangers. You could use one colour for all your work wear, another for leisure clothes, and another for evening clothes. Or, if you share the wardrobe with your partner, you could use different colours for each person's clothes; perhaps dark hangers for yours and light hangers for theirs.

Colour coding books

Colour co-ordinating your books can make your bookcase look very pretty. It's also the easiest place to start if you're just beginning to take your organisation to the next level. If your books are organised like this, rather than by author or subject it can be tricky to find the book you want. To remedy that and to bring your bookshelf to a stratospheric level of organisation, create a spreadsheet with three columns — author, book, colour. Fill in the names of the books on the shelf in the 'book' column, then add the authors. Next, sort the list into alphabetical order based on author. Finally, in the third column write the colour of the spine. Print the sheet and put it somewhere neatly on your bookshelf. Now there's an adaption of the Dewey Decimal System!

Colour coding files

In Chapter 17 on paperwork, I explain how to use colour to organise your paper into files.

Colour coding for kids

Assign a different coloured bin to each child. Use these bins to create a 'tidy up' routine. At the end of the day — maybe just before bedtime, or just after dinner — encourage each child to gather up their toys and put them in their own bin. If that's all that happens, at least the toys are off the floor. Ideally, they can bring that bin and redistribute their toys in their bedrooms or the play room.

In the play room or their bedrooms, you could go one step further and make the toy storage area the same colour as their 'tidy up' bin. This makes it so easy to put toys away because they associate the colour with where their toys live.

DON'T GO CATEGORY CRAZY

If you over-categorise you make retrieval too complicated. Categorisation is a system to help you become more organised. It's designed to make life easier for you, not stress you out. There's a limit to the number of categories you'll remember, so sometimes combining smaller categories together into one bigger one will still keep everything organised and make finding things just as easy. To combine categories successfully, you will need to make sure that the items combined are more alike than unalike.

Remember Monica Geller in *Friends*? She had 11 categories for her towels! The basic category was 'towels' and it was sub-divided into 'everyday', 'guest', 'fancy guest', etc. Eleven sub-categories is definitely category crazy, but you get the idea. Always keep in mind: *easy to find; easy to put away*. If you render retrieval too difficult it defeats the whole purpose of getting organised!

NEVER SAY 'MISCELLANEOUS' AGAIN

There is no such category as 'other', 'general' or 'miscellaneous'. If you start an 'other' category, everything will end up in it. That option usually rears its ugly head when you're starting to get tired. 'Other' then becomes a 'to deal with later' category and all of a sudden you end up with a drawer or shelf full of things that you need to organise and you find yourself back at square one again. Save yourself that trouble and assign a category now.

DECLUTTER

Having gone through your stuff, separated everything out and put it into categories, it's now time to really get stuck in, whittle down the amount of stuff and declutter.

If it's easier for you to combine the categorise and declutter stages, by all means do so. If, when you are categorising, you know immediately that you are going to throw an item away or donate it, do it there and then.

If you haven't started letting things go, now is the time to do so. Armed with what we learned in Chapter 1, we need to keep only items that serve a purpose. Go through each category that you've created and remove anything that does not belong to this space.

Place the item into the box/bag that matches the decision you have made for each item, i.e.

✓ **GENERAL RUBBISH**

✓ **PAPER, PLASTICS**

✓ **DONATE**

✓ **BELONGS ELSEWHERE IN THE HOME**

✓ **BELONGS TO SOMEONE OUTSIDE THE HOME**

It sounds easy enough, but most of the time it's not. Asking yourself some or all of these questions may help as you are trying to figure out if you will keep an item or not:

1 **WHEN DID I LAST USE THIS ITEM?**

2 **HAVE I USED IT IN THE LAST SIX MONTHS? IF NOT, DID I MISS IT OR NEED IT DURING THAT TIME?**

3 **DO I REALLY THINK IT WILL COME BACK INTO FASHION/WILL FIT ONE DAY?**

4 **WOULD SOMEONE ELSE GET BENEFIT FROM THIS NOW?**

5 **IS THIS ITEM REALLY WORTH THE SPACE IT IS TAKING UP? COULD I USE THIS SPACE FOR SOMETHING MORE WORTHWHILE?**

6 **AM I HANGING ONTO THIS ITEM OUT OF GUILT OR FEAR?**

7 **WHAT IS THE WORST THAT COULD HAPPEN IF I LET THIS ITEM GO?**

8 **DO I HAVE THE ORIGINAL AND DO I KNOW WHERE THAT IS?**

9   AM I PLACING SENTIMENTAL VALUE ON TOO MANY THINGS?

10 WILL THE CHILDREN REALLY APPRECIATE ME HANGING ONTO THIS ITEM
    FOR THEM?

11 DO I SEE ANY USE FOR THIS IN THE FUTURE?

12 DO I EVEN LIKE THIS ITEM?

13 DO I REALLY NEED SO MANY COPIES OF THIS?

WHAT ABOUT THE SIX-MONTH RULE?

This is the number one question I am asked and it's not an easy one to answer because it really depends on the amount of stuff you own and the kind of person you are.

Some people love rules and this helps them out enormously. It takes the onus off them to make a decision. If this is the rule, they're happy to go with it and it makes them feel good. Others don't like throwing out the items – usually clothes – that fall into this category and so it causes stress. If you have a closet stuffed to the rafters, or if half your wardrobe is in another room or spends most of the time on the chair in the corner of the bedroom, the six-month rule is more than likely needed here. The level of decluttering you need to do is pretty high.

However, if you have a wardrobe that is relatively okay – it's stuffed, but it's all in one place; you struggle to get at things, but if you really wanted to you could get everything in it – you may have some leeway. And if you have decluttered recently, you probably have some leeway here too.

The choices you make go for everything, from clothes to toys to books. If you have so many items that the space they take up is causing you stress, some of those items need to go in order to give you both physical space and mental peace.

If the pain of having to declutter and get rid of items is greater than the pain of the lack of space, you don't have to get rid of anything.

If this is not how you imagined your wardrobe, spare room or playroom would be like and that is a source of frustration, anger and disappointment, you do something about it. It won't be easy, but you either do or you don't. That comes down to the level of stress this over-stuffed space is causing you. We get comfort from our things, so if it's too hard to let go of items, the comfort of keeping them is greater than your need to have space.

WHAT ABOUT SENTIMENTAL ITEMS?

We put a lot of emphasis on the feelings we get from our possessions. This is particularly true of those that have sentimental meaning. Even I find it difficult to let some things go. And that's why I have, and I insist on all my clients getting, a 'memento' box where they can put anything important to them that they come across during our decluttering sessions. There are some things that are too important to let go of. I understand that.

However, some people can take this to extremes. And it's important to remind yourself that just because you say goodbye to something, you don't say goodbye to the lovely memory or experience that came with it.

SHOULD I ASK A FRIEND TO HELP?

It depends on your friendship! Friends and family mean well and are always there to lend a helping hand. However, getting a satisfactory result depends on the speed at which you can get through clutter. Sometimes, with friends and family, the process can be slower.

I've heard many stories of arguments, too. If you help someone with this, you should go in with a neutral mind: this is not about you or how you would organise things. However, most people don't do that. They may be well intentioned, but differences of opinion often emerge. That's why a professional works better: we have no attachment to you or anything you own.

However, for really tough decisions, or for short stints, a friend can work. Some emotional support may be all you need to let something go. Maybe having a friend or partner with you to reassure you will help you get through this stage more easily.

This is also a lesson in decision-making. It might be easier for you to give away some items to your mother, or your brother, or your friend. But is it easier on them? Do they really need or want these items? Will it put pressure on their space? Will they feel guilty about getting rid of the items?

Ultimately, what stays and what goes is your decision, whether you're with a professional, a friend, or a family member.

The following list of items are easy to throw away and should be done on a regular basis. Don't even give these items your precious time.

✓ **ANYTHING BROKEN THAT CAN'T BE REPAIRED**

✓ **ANYTHING DIRTY THAT IS BEYOND USE EVEN IF CLEANED**

✓ **ANYTHING WITHOUT ITS MATCH – SHOES, SOCKS, GLOVES, SWIMMING ARMBANDS**

✓ **DISCOLOURED PLASTIC CONTAINERS**

✓ **CONTAINERS WITHOUT THEIR LIDS, LIDS WITHOUT THEIR CONTAINERS**

✓ **OLD TIGHTS, POP SOCKS AND UNDERWEAR**

✓ **OLD MAKEUP AND TOILETRIES**

✓ **CLOTHES THAT ARE TOO OLD, BEYOND REPAIR OR TOO SMALL/BIG FOR YOU**

✓ **TOYS OR ANYTHING BELONGING TO THE CHILDREN THAT YOU KNOW THEY WON'T MISS**

✓ **CHILDREN'S DRAWINGS –** you may like to keep ones they drew themselves, but do you need every cartoon or picture they coloured in?

✓ **FINANCIAL RECORDS OLDER THAN SEVEN YEARS –** most financial records can be discarded after seven years, but if you are unsure, check with your bank or solicitor.

✓ **JUNK MAIL –** leaflets on workshops, evening courses, takeaways, cleaners, gardeners, handymen – take note of the contact details if you think you're interested, but get rid of the piece of paper!

✓ **BUSINESS CARDS –** unless you're going to get a business card holder, or file the name and contact information somewhere safe, having it floating around the house is of no use to you or to the person whose card it is. Let it go.

✓ **EMPTY, OUT-OF-DATE DIARIES**

✓ **OLD NEWSPAPERS AND MAGAZINES –** rip out the article(s) you're interested in if you wish, but get rid of the rest of the paper.

✓ **RESEARCH ARTICLES THAT ARE OUT OF DATE**

✓ **EMPTY ENVELOPES –** when you open your post, put the envelope in your recycling bin.

✓ **CARDBOARD BOXES –** especially boxes from purchases of technology – you need the cables, the guarantee and the instruction manual, so take them out, file them away and get rid of the box.

✓ **PAPER SHOPPING BAGS AND PLASTIC BAGS –** having a handful is handy when you need a spare bag. But you don't need a collection of them. Reuse them or recycle them.

✓ **BROKEN PENS, STAPLERS, SCISSORS, FOLDERS OR ANY STATIONERY THAT DOESN'T WORK**

✓ **OLD AND BATTERED PLASTIC FOLDERS, POLY POCKETS OR DOCUMENT WALLETS**

✓ **PEN LIDS WITHOUT THE CORRESPONDING PEN**

✓ **EMPTY CD CASES**

✓ **OLD BATTERIES, BROKEN LIGHT BULBS, OLD PHONES, OLD PHONE CHARGERS, RIPPED WIRING**

SOME MORE TIPS

Don't know? Don't sweat it!

As with the categorise stage, if you really, really can't decide what to do with an item, leave it to one side. Don't get bogged down or start beating yourself up over your indecision. Just leave it and move on.

Start tough!

In the categorise stage, I recommended pulling out the things that are easiest to categorise. This was to help you get started; to make the process a little easier and to encourage you on your way.

Now, however, I recommend the opposite. Just picking out the easy things to make a decision about may ease you in gently, but it's just delaying the inevitable.

I suggest leaving the easier things until the end and forcing yourself to make decisions on the harder things first. Why? Because you're going to get tired. When you get tired, you're just going to say 'forget this' and give up. But if you get through all the hard decisions first, then just as you're starting to get tired and bored, you'll only have the easier stuff to go. You'll be able to get through these things quicker and so will stay motivated to stick with the decluttering to the end.

You're playing a blinder, but there are some things you just can't part with. It's now or never!

Eliminate or hibernate — *Get rid of it now, or place the item(s) in the attic or basement for six months. If you haven't missed it or needed to use it at the end of six months, I think it's safe to let it go.*

Need or impede — *Do you really need it, or is it going to impede how you use this space? Do you really need three sets of cutlery? Fifteen kitchen whisks? Three copies of the same magazine from January 1980? Is this object going to get in your way?*

Enjoy or destroy — *You're either going to get use and enjoyment out of this object or you're not. Pulling it out from the back of the wardrobe, struggling on a decision and then putting it back where you found it is not getting use or enjoyment out of it. Time to destroy it! Drastic, maybe, but we're really going for it here!*

Own or moan — *Are you going to take ownership of this item, use it, share it, enjoy it? Or are you going to keep it but moan about it and your lack of space?*

You can't complain about lack of space if your decisions always result in keeping more items than space allows.

Debate or donate

While you're having an inner debate, remember that it's always your decision. You can keep something, or you can let it go. Remember the importance of donations. Someone may need what you don't a lot more than you need to keep it.

WHAT IS THIS PROCESS BRINGING UP FOR YOU?

Getting rid of some items can bring up a lot of emotions and memories. It can be a real journey, looking over your past and what you thought would be your future; and looking towards your future as it is now. It can cause utter panic to let go of items. Which can then result in anger with yourself.

✓ **WHY CAN'T I DO THIS?**

✓ **WHAT'S WRONG WITH ME?**

✓ **I FEEL AWFUL.**

✓ **I FEEL LIKE CRYING.**

✓ **I CAN'T THINK STRAIGHT.**

✓ **I'M NOT GOING TO DO THIS.**

✓ **I CAN'T DO IT.**

✓ **I DON'T WANT TO DO IT.**

✓ **EVERYONE ELSE CAN DO IT, WHY CAN'T I?**

How does this line of questioning help? Beating yourself up is not going to make a difference to your physical space but it will damage your mental space. You really need to bring your A game here.

Sometimes it's good to have a cry. Cry for five minutes, then get back to it. Let it out but don't let it stop you. Then focus on the task at hand. Do it a bit at a time. Remember your time limit. And then finish up.

Once you're done, look at your calendar and decide when you will declutter again. If you can declutter again the next day or in two days' time, so much the better. I promise you, if you do it regularly, it gets easier. Try me on this, I dare you.

It's awful the first time, not so good the second time, and then slightly easier the third time. If you declutter regularly, you get used to making decisions and get used to the feelings that come up. This can help you in many areas of your life. But only if you do it regularly. It will stay hard if you only dip in and out every now and then.

Life might be telling you to start confronting something. Respond to that, don't resist it. Respond with love, not with frustration.

WRITING

Writing is a great way to sort out our feelings and emotions. So if throwing things away is troubling you, it might help to write about it.

✓ **WHAT EMOTION ARE YOU EXPERIENCING?**

✓ **HAVE YOU EXPERIENCED THIS EMOTION BEFORE?**

✓ **WHEN WAS THAT?**

✓ **WHAT DOES THIS ITEM REPRESENT TO YOU?**

✓ **WHAT MEMORY DOES IT HOLD?**

✓ **HOW WOULD YOU FEEL WITHOUT IT?**

TALKING

Talking to a therapist can also be hugely helpful.

At the end of the day, this is an exercise in letting go and change, neither of which most humans like. It's not about your stuff – your feelings about your things are merely symptoms of something else going on.

MEDITATING

Meditation puts the brakes on. It offers a few moments of peace and calm. You then carry that peace and calm with you as you start into the activities of the day. Don't be like a kitten chasing its tail – an adult cat doesn't do that; it has learned to sit and curl its tail around. So stop running around in circles. Sit and assess.

Just like organising, you may think you don't have time for meditation. However, it is exactly when you think you don't have time to organise or to meditate that you need to do it. And it's precisely because of this perceived lack of time that you need to do it.

It's all just too much. There's too much going on. Too much stuff, too many demands on your time, too many people talking, too much information, another text pings on your phone, a bill arrives through the post box.

Enough.

Why do you think some people clean and organise when times get tough? Because it gives a feeling of taking back control. Cleaning and organising can be like a meditation to some people. They forget everything else and polish the mirrors or file paperwork. There can be a trance-like state to this type of work.

Whether you get to that point or not is irrelevant. The point is that when there's too much going on, you can halt it for a few moments. Sit and breathe for five minutes. And when you've organised your time and your environment so that they work with you, you may find that you're feeling more in control. Your situation may not have changed, but your attitude to it has.

Restarts aren't just for 1 January or for Mondays. Restarts can happen at any time. Step out of the high-octane pace of life for a few seconds. Let your brain catch up, rest and assess. Then go again with a new approach.

ORGANISE

When you've categorised and decluttered, you know exactly what you own. Therefore, you can organise a good home for things because you can see exactly how much space all your items take up.

Organising homes for your things does not equal new storage solutions. At this stage, *organising is using the* furniture, *space* and, indeed, the storage *you already have*. You're putting items away again, but using the space in a more effective and efficient way. Storage solutions – if they're needed at all – will come later. Generally this is where people get confused. You don't always need storage solutions. Organisation means using your current space well. This is sometimes enhanced with storage, but it can and should be done without that expense. Having a storage solution doesn't mean your home is organised – often the storage solutions are full of clutter. Whereas you can achieve good organisation without having storage.

At this point, your drawers, cabinets and shelves are empty and what you have decided to keep is waiting to be re-homed. We'll organise all these items now and make best use of your space. We'll add storage later.

FUNCTIONS OF THE HOME

One of the keys to becoming organised is managing the function of a room. Traditionally, a home has:

- ✓ **KITCHEN, FOR COOKING**

- ✓ **LIVING ROOM, FOR RELAXING/ENTERTAINING**

- ✓ **DINING ROOM, FOR EATING/ENTERTAINING**

- ✓ **BATHROOM, FOR BATHING/SHOWERING**

- ✓ **BEDROOMS, FOR SLEEPING**

However, over the years, social and economic developments have resulted in a lot of changes to the functions of a home.

Many people work from home now, and they need an office to work in. With the amount of paperwork that arrives through our letterbox each day, most of us need a makeshift office at the best of times anyway. At the very least, virtually everyone has a laptop and probably a printer.

Children have more toys, DVDs and game consoles than ever before, so a lot of families dedicate an entire room to a toy room/play room.

Many young couples bought their first apartment during the Celtic Tiger years, and just as they were getting married and starting a family, the bottom fell out of the housing market, they went into negative equity and found they couldn't afford to move into the three-bed semi-detached as they had always planned. So whole families are now growing up in small apartments.

Many more people than before are renting their home. Renting comes with a lot of conditions. Perhaps you can't get an unfurnished home, so you're stuck with the furniture someone else chose and which may not meet your needs. Or perhaps you aren't allowed to put shelving on the walls.

So is it any wonder that any space in a home is precious? With limited space, the functions of rooms are frequently merged together and this results in a lot of disorganisation. There is rarely such a thing as a 'spare room' anymore. It's full of things you can't fit into the attic, or would fit into the attic if you had one!

There is no problem with one room having two functions, but two should ideally be the maximum. An open-plan kitchen extends to a dining and living space that also contains some toys. A guest room doubles as an office. In dual-purpose rooms, functions must be clearly separated to work well. In order to keep the function of a room and, by extension, the organisation of a room in check, you need to learn how to create zones in your home.

The art of creating zones is keeping similar objects together (a category) *near* where you use them. Good organisation means that items are easy to retrieve and easy to put away. If they are near where you would use them, that will happen. For example, you might put your crockery in the press above the dishwasher so it makes it easier to unload the dishwasher. You could keep your DVDs in a drawer under the television unit so that they are nearby when you want to watch one. You might keep a box of tissues in the hallway so you can grab one as you run out of the door each morning.

These are all zones: *areas picked out and planned with the specific aim of having an object in a certain location exactly when you need it.* Zones suit the function of the room and/or our use of an item.

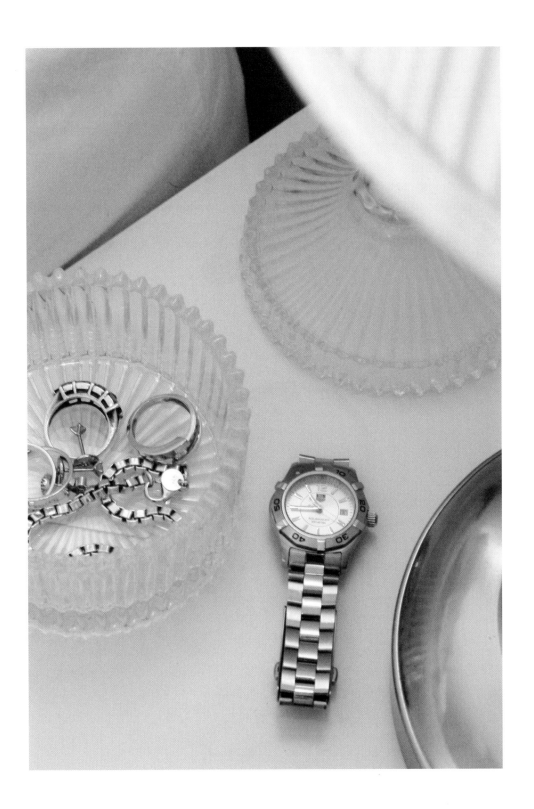

Creating zones can be done on a large or a small scale. On a large scale, you will zone an entire room. For example, an open-plan living room with a seated area for the TV and toys for the kids could be zoned by using the furniture and a rug to indicate the boundaries in the room. The furniture indicates 'no toys beyond this point' and all toys are kept in a little nook behind the couch.

On a small scale, you can zone an individual drawer, shelf, cabinet, even container. A bookshelf could hold books, DVDs, computer games and consoles, framed photos and ornaments. Zoning that bookshelf would involve placing all the books together on one shelf, perhaps two. Whether or not the shelves with the books are full, a separate shelf is dedicated to DVDs and computer games. The top shelf can be zoned for photos and another shelf zoned for consoles and other technology.

There are hundreds of zones that can be created in your home to maximise the organisation of your space. Below are some popular and useful zones that can be replicated in your home.

STATIONERY ZONE

We love our stationery! We have a ton of it, but it's scattered everywhere throughout the house and we just can't find the scissors or Sellotape when we need it. So we need to create a zone.

If you have a home office, you might want to put the majority of your stationery there. However, whether you have a home office or not, I generally find that you need small stationery zones in the kitchen, too, and perhaps in each of the kids' bedrooms.

CLEANING AND LAUNDRY SUPPLIES ZONE

Most of us already have this zone set up – it's usually under the sink. However, sometimes under the sink can be a large space with no clear definition, and we generally just dump things on top of each other. You may also have some laundry products in a utility or laundry room. Keeping track of what we have and what we might need can be difficult. In that case, bring all the products together. Categorise them according to their job – laundry/dusting/bathroom, etc. – and put them near where you will use them. Use storage containers to hold the products together in their new zone. Or perhaps add some shelving under the sink so as to maximise the amount of useful space under there.

MAKEUP AND TOILETRIES ZONE

These categories are usually either in the bedroom or the bathroom and very often in both. You have your makeup in the bedroom but you prefer the lighting in the bathroom, so you end up going back and forth between rooms. Or you end up bringing your products into the bathroom, and because they have no designated place, they accumulate on your bathroom counters and shelving.

So make a decision. Where do you use these things? If it's in the bathroom but you don't have the space for them, ask yourself if you're keeping too much. Could you declutter things a bit? Could you add more shelving on the walls, or a small cabinet under the basin? Or how about some hanging storage for the back of the door? All these suggestions may help you bring your products into the area where you use them; and in doing so, you create a zone.

You might also want to create smaller zone pockets. For instance, if you go to the gym, you might like to organise a wash bag and place that in your gym bag ready for use. Or you might like to organise a small makeup bag and put it in your handbag for work. These are also zones – you're placing items next to where you'll use them!

HOUSEHOLD DOCUMENTS ZONE

Every home needs to sort this zone out. From passports and birth certs to manuals and school information, there is a lot of paperwork in our lives, and keeping it in shape will really help our stress levels.

I think having a folder or expanding file near the kitchen is a good spot for a household administration zone. Place papers that you need regular and quick access to in there and create a little Home Management folder for yourself. However, if you have a home office, I would recommend filing as many papers as possible there.

OUTDOOR GEAR AND ACCESSORIES ZONE

Whether you are rushing the kids to school or setting off for a family picnic, there are some items that it would be really handy to have to hand: hats, scarves, gloves, sunglasses, Wellington boots, coats, shoes, raingear, tissues etc.

A great zone for these items is in the hallway. You might have the luxury of a mud room, but if you don't, never fear. If you can't keep all these items together in one spot, place them according to family member in their bedrooms. You will be creating a smaller zone in each bedroom.

When we're getting organised we talk about giving 'homes' to things. I prefer to give items a job to do. Every shelf, every drawer, every console, press, cabinet, container, bin, basket, even paperclip gets some organising job to do. If you do nothing else, do this!

Make your furniture and storage work for you; give everything a job to do. For example, you have four containers on two shelves in the kitchen: one container has the job of holding tea bags; the next holds coffee; the third holds snacks; the fourth holds confectionery. The shelves themselves have a job to do: the bottom shelf holds the tea and coffee containers and the top shelf holds the snacks and confectionery.

In the guest room which doubles as an office, there are two cupboards. The job of one cupboard is to hold office paraphernalia. The other cupboard is excess storage space for home supplies – nothing office-related allowed.

In the office cupboard itself, there are six shelves and, yes, each one has a job. The top two hold business magazines and research papers. The next two hold office stationery and supplies. One shelf holds technology and multimedia and the bottom one holds files.

Everything is assigned a job. *Items are arranged as per their job.* From something as small as a basket to something as big as a wardrobe shelf, everything has a job. Why? Because if you don't do that, people will dump anything anywhere. An organised division of labour makes it clear to everyone what does and does not belong in a given space.

ACCESS

When you approach your space – whether that space is a container, your wardrobe or your garage – what is the access like? The system of organisation will stay in place if you can get to things easily. If you are fighting your way to get to something, then when it comes putting things away, you won't bother; you'll drop things as close as possible to the destination. To maintain organisation, that just won't do. When placing items back into cabinets, onto shelves and into drawers, it's always done in priority order. The item that goes into a space first will be the least used item. Items you need daily should be within arm's reach.

Due to a lack of space, sometimes we need to place items in front of something else. If you do place items in front of each other, arrange smaller items to the front of taller ones so that you can see everything.

If an item needs to go in front of another, make sure there's only one item in front; two at the absolute maximum. Make sure the items to the front are very easy to pull out in order to get behind. Make the pathway clear and easy.

For hard-to-reach areas, buy a foot stool and for dark areas, a light.

LIGHTING

Speaking of light, I find one big contributing factor to disorganisation is a lack of good lighting. Whether it's the garage, attic, under the stairs, or a deep kitchen cupboard, making sure there's good light coming into the area will help you keep it tidy. It's one thing to be constricted due to a lack of space, it's another to not be able to see any space at all. Shine a light on your situation!

HIGH SHELVES AND DEEP DRAWERS

Things that we don't use often are arranged on the top shelves in any room and at the back of deep presses and shelves. If you have a lot of presses up high in your home, consider them primarily as a place for storage. These hard-to-reach areas are like an addition to your garage or attic and should be for Christmas decorations, out-of-season clothes, gifts you received that you can't give away but you won't use, good crystal and china that you want to protect. Make sure you have a stool to reach high locations; again, focus on ease of retrieval.

WATCH YOUR HABITS

Remember, we always organise to allow for easy retrieval in future. When you are organising items in your space, it's important to keep the things you use most often within easy reach. This is when the use of an object takes precedence over available space.

For example, if you declutter your hallway, you may decide that when you arrive in from work, you'd like to 'home' your handbag on a nearby shelf. However, the shelf is a little out of reach. Yes the space is available, but it just wouldn't work. You won't walk in the door each night and stretch up to the shelf to put your bag away. You'll fire it into the hallway like you do every night. Similarly, when you're rushing out of the door in the morning, it would be a right pain to have to reach up and grab the bag. Remember to be aware of your habits. Wouldn't it be easier just to hang it up on a hook right inside the door?

New 'homes' need to be very easy. If there's a change, it can't be too far off what you and the family were doing already. If there's any effort at all, items just won't be put away and you will lose the organisation.

You can't organise your home without taking your existing habits into consideration. If those existing habits need to change with organisation, make sure you're comfortable with that. Otherwise, change the organisation and find another 'home'.

A note on hallways

This is the area of your home with the most traffic. People and their things coming in and out. In some homes this area leads into the utility or mud room.

It's always the same collection of items here: gifts bought for events, which will be taken out; donations en route to the charity shop; sports bags left between training sessions; bicycle helmets; shoes; and coats … many, many coats.

For items that are in transit and will be moving out shortly, place a large basket near the door. This will tidy up the hallway and stop the sprawl. Hooks for bags, coats and helmets keep items off the floor and off the banisters.

While solutions can be placed to catch the main culprits, this space is rife with poor tidying habits. It is a change of habit that will make a real difference here: bringing our things all the way to the relevant room the minute we arrive and not just dropping and leaving them in the hall.

Any storage you add here must be a solution for the most common items first. To ensure the smooth running of your home, make sure you are not giving vital hallway storage to items of lower priority.

HOLD BACK

When you start to organise and reduce some of your clutter, space will start to emerge. Thoughts of 'Yippee!', 'Thank God!', 'Let's put this here, and that there' follow very quickly! So hold back! Just because there's space doesn't mean you have to use it. You don't have to fill every square inch of free space. Items need to be arranged more mindfully and methodically.

You use space if it allows you to keep categories together within a zone. You use space if it makes sense for your habits and how you use the room. Leaving a few open areas in rooms, presses and on shelves makes the area seem less cluttered and by extension more airy, bright and visually calming.

You also need to *allow for growth*. You will acquire new things. So when you place items in their new homes, make sure the home you assign has enough room if you ever need to add more.

It sounds more complicated and a longer process than it actually is. I like to think of it as like putting together a jigsaw. Technically, if you wanted you could put whatever pieces you like together and force them to slot in with each other. But it would look a mess and would never work. Done properly, however, each piece of a jigsaw belongs to another piece and they fit perfectly together to create a beautiful picture.

PUTTING IT ALL TOGETHER

When deciding where you are going to home your things, sit down and plan it out. Look at the space you have in a room in comparison to what you want to house there. We have finished categorising and decluttering our things and we are down to what we really need, love and use.

You can only effectively organise when you know what your categories are and the size of them. You then compare the size of the categories to the size of the available space and match them up in a way that suits your habits. This requires some thought and planning. There's an art to this organisation!

1 **ASSESS THE CATEGORIES**: Take an inventory of the things you are going to keep. It doesn't have to be a perfect list, just a quick totting-up of the categories you have created.

2 **ASSESS THE SPACE**: Now look at the area(s) you are going to arrange your things into. What space do you have? What drawers, presses, wall space is there available to you? Make a list of those too.

3 **MATCH**: Now match up and plan which items are going to go into which place. Draw or write down what homes you are going to assign to what items. To help, ask yourself: next time I need this, where would I be? (this establishes the room or space in the room); and what would I need it for? (this establishes what other items or category/ies it might live with/ beside.)

4 ORGANISE: Put your plan into action. For example:

You are organising your living room. The following categories have been created:

- ✓ DVDS
- ✓ BOOKS
- ✓ ORNAMENTS
- ✓ CANDLES
- ✓ PHOTOS

- ✓ EMPTY PHOTO FRAMES
- ✓ PHOTO ALBUMS
- ✓ BOARD GAMES
- ✓ ELECTRONIC WIRING FOR GAMES CONSOLE, TV, PHONES, DVD PLAYER AND CAMERAS

The space available is as follows:

- ✓ BOOKCASE WITH SIX SHELVES
- ✓ SMALLER BOOKCASE WITH THREE OPEN SHELVES AND A CUPBOARD WITH THREE SHELVES
- ✓ DVD/CD TOWER WITH 60 SLOTS
- ✓ TV UNIT WITH TWO DRAWERS
- ✓ FIREPLACE MANTELPIECE
- ✓ WALL SPACE

You decide to arrange your items as follows:

LARGE BOOKCASE (SIX SHELVES)	→	books and ornaments
SMALL BOOKCASE (TWO OF THE THREE SHELVES)	→	books
SMALL BOOKCASE (CUPBOARD)	→	stock of candles, photo albums, empty photo frames
DVD/CD TOWER	→	DVDs
TV UNIT (FIRST DRAWER)	→	electronic wiring
TV UNIT (SECOND DRAWER)	→	board games
MANTELPIECE	→	ornaments, candles
WALL SPACE	→	photos

But what happens if you find that the home you chose for a certain category of items doesn't fit everything? After planning it all out, when you got down to arranging your things in their new homes, you discovered the reality is this:

✓ **THE DVDS DON'T FIT IN THE CD TOWER.**

✓ **THERE ARE MORE BOOKS THAN THE SPACE ON THE TWO BOOKCASES ALLOWS.**

✓ **ALL THE PHOTO ALBUMS WON'T FIT ON THE SMALLER BOOKCASE.**

✓ **AND EVEN THOUGH THE ELECTRONIC WIRING FITS IN THE DRAWER IN THE TV UNIT, IT STILL LOOKS JUMBLED UP.**

Never fear! Keep breathing. This is where people start thinking, 'Nothing is ever going to fit,' and just give up. It's like a jigsaw, remember, so you might have to move things around.

✓ **THE DVDS.** Abandon the CD tower and try the second drawer of the TV unit instead. This is in keeping with our zones: you use the TV to watch the DVDs.

✓ **THE BOOKS.** Assuming that you absolutely cannot throw out or donate any more of your books (are you really sure?), take a look around. Do you have enough wall space for another bookcase? What sort of books are you keeping in the living room? Are there cookery books that could go to the kitchen? Are there children's books that could go to their bedrooms? 'But wouldn't I be splitting up a category?' you say. No, you wouldn't: you are merely creating a 'books' category in your kitchen and a 'books' category in your children's bedrooms. And the bonus is that they are located in a space that complements them, i.e. zones. Where else but in the kitchen would you need your cookery books?

✓ **THE PHOTO ALBUMS.** Now that you've moved some of the books to other rooms, could more photo albums fit on the bookcase? Do the photo albums also warrant looking at buying that other bookcase we spoke about?

✓ **THE WIRING.** This requires a storage solution. They are organised, but to streamline them you need some storage. In the meantime, be happy you have finally found one home for all your wiring. You got them all together, got rid of the wiring that didn't work and found a home. That's the hardest job done; getting better storage is the fun part!

When items don't fit where you hoped they would, don't panic. Look at the next shelf/drawer/cabinet and see if they will fit there. Items will still be near each other and near where they are used. Storage solutions will also help in this instance, and we'll discuss that later.

FINISHING TOUCHES

I always find when I'm decluttering with a client that there is one item that follows us around. We come across it during the categorising stage and a client will not know exactly what it is but knows they don't want to throw it out. Or they know what it is but are unsure how to categorise it. So we leave this item to one side initially. When we get to the stage where we are organising items back into their new homes, this one little thing will still be knocking about!

Trust me, you will have the pleasure of the acquaintance of a pesky item like this during your own decluttering session. It's at this organising stage that you really need to decide what you are going to do with it. *You need to name it and home it. Or get rid of it.*

Now that you have re-arranged your things, you've almost finished your decluttering session. Now we complete the task's circle and move on to the clear-up. It's broken into three parts:

1 TIDY UP

2 STORAGE

3 LABELLING

TIDY UP

When you decide to organise a room or area, you have to factor in time to clean up at the end. Pulling things out and rearranging will cause some debris and a lot of dust. If it's just left like that, it will take away from all the good organising you have just spent time doing. A good tidy after you put things back will not only force you to make sure that everything, no matter how small, gets a home, it also helps hold the organisation in place until you finalise the project with storage solutions.

Rather than putting the last item away and thinking, 'Well, that's all I can do now until I get some storage,' tidying up actually makes the room usable, even without storage. If you need to buy storage, getting it as quickly as possible will ensure that the room doesn't go back to its old ways, so do prioritise it on your schedule.

There will always be little items that fall out during decluttering, for example hair clips, coins, paper clips, pens, buttons, batteries, empty CD/DVD/sunglasses cases, scraps of paper with telephone numbers on them, seed packets, bits of ribbon, etc. You have to deal with them in order to finish off the room. All these things need homes. It's at this stage that people often give up. These items are too small to bother with, or they'll be dealt with next time.

But it is these very small items that cause clutter in the first place. All these tiny items have no homes. If you really want one of those lovely, well-organised, bright and airy, spacious rooms that you're always admiring, then you are going to have to find a home for every one of these annoying little things. They do belong somewhere. Even if it is just in the bin!

Once you find a home for all these little things, they won't annoy you again. Next time you find a stray hair clip or a lone button, you'll know where to put it.

You will also have uncovered these items:

- ITEMS THAT BELONG TO OTHER ROOMS: Take items that you have decided belong to other rooms and put them away properly. Don't just dump them on the floor or a cabinet top and say you'll get back to them later. You won't. Put them away properly now. If you are reluctant to put items into other rooms because the other rooms are also full of clutter, do so anyway. Yes, these other rooms may need work, but the item in your hand belongs in this room, not in the room you have just decluttered.

- ITEMS FOR DONATION: If you haven't done so already, place the items that you have designated for donations in a box or plastic bag and label it. Put the box/bag in your hallway or in the car boot. Don't leave it in the newly organised room. Now that you have finally decided to part with certain items, you need to keep moving them out of the house. So get them out towards the door. Put 'Donate items' on your to-do list and schedule in time to do just that!

- ITEMS THAT BELONG TO OTHER PEOPLE: If you have found items that were lent to you years ago and you still have them, you need to move them out of your house now. Place them all in a box and put a Post-it or label on each item with the name of the person each item has to go back to.

- GENERAL RUBBISH: Take general rubbish to the bin and put paper and plastic rubbish in the recycling.

In summary, here's a tidy-up checklist:

- ✓ **PUT DONATION BOXES/BAGS IN THE HALL.**

- ✓ **RUBBISH AND RECYCLING BAGS TO THE BINS.**

- ✓ **RELOCATE ITEMS THAT BELONG ELSEWHERE.**

- ✓ **MAKE A LIST OF ITEMS/CATEGORIES THAT REQUIRE STORAGE.**

- ✓ **MAKE A LIST OF ANY DIY REQUIRED IN THE ROOM.**

- ✓ **A QUICK DUST OR VACUUM TO STRAIGHTEN UP THE ROOM, PUT AWAY YOUR DECLUTTERING TOOLS AND CLEANING PRODUCTS AND ...**

- ✓ **TA DAH! YOU'RE DONE!**

STORAGE

When we want to get organised, what's the first thing we do? We go out and we buy storage that we think is going to solve the problem. However, the new storage products won't fit where we had hoped to put them. Or they won't hold everything we wanted to put into them. We've wasted our money and the product goes to waste, becoming another piece of clutter around the home. Oh, the irony!

There's a common assumption that all we need is more space and more storage. Clients often say, 'I just need a bigger house.' Unfortunately, what we tend to do when we get more space is to fill it. It's great that you don't have to look at so much clutter any more, but can you find everything? Is the clutter simply hidden behind a door or in a container? If you accumulate even more, will you be able to put those things away?

Getting organised is not as simple as putting a few items in a container and – hey presto – you're organised. As we've seen, organisation involves an awareness of your habits, how you use things, how you use your home and why. Storage does bring organisation together and streamlines space. It gives homes to all our things and makes it very easy to access everything. However, it's not always the answer. Another container, box, or even an extension can be just another place to dump things. It's not the storage that solves your issue. Sometimes you have to remove the storage in order to achieve organisation. If there's one too many places to dump things, then removing the storage option is often your answer.

A coat rack in a hallway covered in coats can get untidy quickly. When you declutter the coats, you might find you're only keeping two or three, all of which could go elsewhere. But what will you do with the coat rack now, you ask. Remove it. Remove the option to dump coats there. Remove the option that clutters up your hallway. *Change the habit.* And encourage family members to put their coats elsewhere.

The kids' small desk in the kitchen or living room was placed there to allow them to paint or draw or do homework. However, they usually end up doing all that at the kitchen table. If they do it at all. The small desk, which is never used, is covered in scribbles and random bits of paper and clutter. You're reluctant to remove it because they might use it one day. But the reason they might use it no longer exists. It doesn't work. It's attracting clutter and creating a mess. So get rid of this 'solution'.

When I put organisation into a house, I learn about your way of life and your behaviour. Based on what you tell me, I place solutions to catch everything that comes with living that life. Or I remove them. It's recognising that when something works, don't change it; make it better. It's questioning and challenging how and why you currently choose to treat some items or use some spaces in certain ways.

If it was as easy as getting a box, we'd all have beautifully organised homes. But it's not the box, it's the behaviour.

DOING A STORAGE AUDIT

I can completely understand why we have accumulated things as we have. Following the scarcity of the World Wars, we consumed as much as we could as a kind of security blanket should another war happen. This trend was passed on from generation to generation and so materialism grew.

The idea that the more we have, the happier we'll be leads to more and more spending. We want to keep up with the neighbours. We want to be an early adopter of the next big thing. We want everything the blogger has. We are always searching for more. However, homes full of stuff, most of which goes unused, result in anxiety, stress and depression, not happiness.

The trend may be shifting. 'Stuffocation', a term coined by trend forecaster James Wallman, is the idea that modern society is moving away from believing that more *things* make us happy and toward the idea that *experiences* make us feel more fulfilled. We can actually live with very little. Our wellbeing comes from our relationships, our health, hobbies, challenges.

The amount of material possessions we have nowadays is at an all-time high. The growth in consumption over the last 50 years puts a major strain on our environment. From food to makeup to cigarettes to toys, the amount of stuff we buy is enormous. It's a waste of our money and a literal waste that's affecting the environment.

When you start decluttering, doing an audit of the storage you already have to make sure you use what you have is a very good place to start. To reduce waste, donating, recycling, selling items and only buying what you need always helps.

RECYCLING AND UPCYCLING

If you can recycle or upcycle your current storage, you get maximum use out of the product, help the planet and, of course, help your pocket. It can also encourage you to get creative.

There are hundreds of DIY videos on YouTube that show you how to create storage and upcycle. We all keep shoe boxes to help us organise our stuff. Here are just a few other examples:

- MAGAZINE RACKS for baking trays or pot lids

- CLOTHES PEGS for wires

- ICE CUBE TRAYS for earrings/rings

- CUTLERY TRAYS for makeup or (standing upright with hooks) for jewellery

- PAPER TOWEL HOLDER for black plastic bag dispenser

- BASKET underneath a desk for computer wires/extension leads

- PLANT POTS for cutlery

- CANVAS SHOE HOLDER for paper/stationery/files

As you declutter, containers you were using will empty. I always keep the spare storage to one side until the very end. If you're doing this, don't leave storage scattered around the house. Pile it up together in one place, perhaps a spare room or the garage. Use old storage as much as possible and only throw it out if it's broken. Donate it if it's not going to be used.

HOW TO SHOP FOR STORAGE

If you do need new storage, this is when you move from the pain of decluttering to the fun of organisation. There's a knack to shopping for storage. First, ask yourself:

✓ **DO I REALLY NEED IT?**

✓ **WILL IT REALLY FIT WHERE I THINK IT WILL?**

✓ **WILL IT LOOK GOOD?**

✓ **WHAT AM I GOING TO USE IT FOR?**

✓ **WILL EVERYTHING I'M THINKING OF FIT INSIDE?**

✓ **WOULD SOME OTHER SOLUTION WORK BETTER?**

Then:

1   **MAKE A LIST**

2   **MEASURE AND MEASURE AGAIN**

3   **ALLOW FOR GROWTH**

STEP 1. MAKE A LIST

Most people, whether they're shopping for food or birthday presents, will put together a quick list of what they think they need. So with storage you'd think you'd do the same, right? Wrong!

A traditional shopping list details what we need, and we often think the same way for our storage solutions. But when you create a list for storage, instead of listing the storage you think you want to buy, list the items you need to store.

Let's say you have decluttered your bedroom. The old you is thinking that you'd like to get some hangers, some hooks, a shoe rack and a jewellery box. But how about thinking about it like this instead? After organising your wardrobe and taking an inventory, you folded some clothes, but you would like to hang:

- 3 skirts

- 8 pairs of trousers

- 6 dresses

- 9 T-shirts

- 3 shirts

You also have a slight shoe problem. When you counted them you had:

- 5 pairs of knee-high boots
- 4 pairs runners
- 6 pairs sandals
- 4 pairs wedge-heel sandals

- 18 pairs high heels
- 8 pairs ankle boots
- 1 pair flip-flops
- 1 pair slippers

- 1 pair golf shoes
- 1 pair hiking boots
- 3 pairs pumps

And you'd like to organise the following better:

- 10 handbags
- 3 hats
- Jewellery – consisting of earrings, rings, two watches and lots of necklaces

The new organised you goes to the shops with a list that looks like this:

✓ **29 HANGERS**

✓ **SOLUTION FOR 53+ PAIRS OF SHOES**

✓ **ENOUGH HOOKS OR A HANGING STORAGE SOLUTION TO ALLOW FOR 10+ HANDBAGS**

✓ **HAT BOXES FOR EACH HAT, OR ONE BIG ENOUGH TO HOLD ALL THREE**

✓ **A JEWELLERY SOLUTION THAT ALLOWS FOR LOTS OF HANGING SPACE/HOOKS**

The shopping list details the items you need a solution for, not the solution itself. The exception here is the hangers, of course. Hangers are the solution and the only solution. So of course it's more efficient to list hangers and the number required rather than write all the articles of clothes that need them.

By creating a list in this way, you are more focused on what you need and less likely to impulse buy. Which saves you money.

GETTING
ORGANISED IS
NOT AS SIMPLE
AS PUTTING A
FEW ITEMS IN A
CONTAINER.

Now you are going to be much more specific with what you buy. You are more detailed with your instructions to yourself. You are going to be on the lookout, not just for any old bit of storage, but storage that can actually hold what you need it to hold. You are less likely to buy something that *might* work and more likely to get storage that suits your space and your needs.

STEP 2. MEASURE AND MEASURE AGAIN

You have an idea of places in your home where you would like to add storage. Now you need to make sure that the designated home fits the new storage. Measure the area in question before you buy anything to make absolutely sure that you buy the right sized storage for your chosen area.

✓ IF YOU'RE LOOKING FOR A BOOKCASE – MEASURE THE WALL

✓ IF YOU'RE LOOKING FOR CONTAINERS TO GO IN A KITCHEN CABINET – MEASURE THE DEPTH OF THE CABINET

✓ IF YOU'D LIKE TO ADD BASKETS TO SHELVES IN THE BATHROOM – MEASURE THE SHELVES

✓ IF YOU'D LIKE TO ADD BOXES TO THE TOP OF YOUR WARDROBES – MEASURE THE HEIGHT, WIDTH AND DEPTH AVAILABLE

STEP 3. ALLOW FOR GROWTH

When you are choosing storage, always bear in mind that the amount of stuff you own will more than likely increase. Until you get around to your next decluttering session, you want to have storage that will allow for and hold any increase in stuff. So, while you only have 53 pairs of shoes *now*, you might just end up buying those Kurt Geiger heels you saw at half price. It's important to recognise your shoe addiction.

An organised storage shopping list might look like this.

SPACE	SOLUTIONS FOR:	AREAS FOR STORAGE	DIMENSIONS		
			HEIGHT	WIDTH	DEPTH
MASTER WARDROBE	29 hangers	Bed drawers			
	53+ pairs of shoes	Left-hand wall			
	Hat boxes for each hat, or one big enough to hold all three	Upper wardrobe shelves			
	A jewellery solution that allows for lots of hanging space/hooks				

SPACE	SOLUTIONS FOR:	AREAS FOR STORAGE	DIMENSIONS		
			HEIGHT	WIDTH	DEPTH
KITCHEN	Cooking oils currently on counter	Under sink	24.5cm	24.5cm	24.5cm
	Cloths and sponges	Upper cabinet above cooker	22cm	81cm	26cm
	Snacks and confectionery	Drawers under microwave	14.5cm	48cm	44.5cm
	Tupperware				

So next time you need storage, use your own version of this storage shopping list template and get storage that works for the items and fits the space.

LABELLING

There is no point having a lovely organised space, with great storage, if you are still unsure what's inside. And even if you know what's inside, does everyone in the family? Once you have cut through clutter and started to organise new 'homes', labelling will help.

Very often we are sure that we are going to remember, but we don't. There are new homes for things and new ways of using the space. It might be just one step too far to expect our brains to remember every single change. So let's help it out.

Even the most organised of spaces can be brought up another level with a label. As we discussed in Chapter 1, organisation takes the burden off your brain. *Labels completely remove any thinking* from the way you use your stuff. You might remember what's in each box, but with a label you don't even have to bother doing that. The label is the reminder. It does the work for you. It's easy to find things and easy to put them away. No mess, no time wasting. Labels don't have to stay for ever, just until the new systems become second nature. Just remember not to over-do labels. For some containers it's blatantly obvious what's inside. Labels are gorgeous, but like everything, use in moderation and be organised in their use!

Standard labels
If you're stuck for time or money, grab a plain label and a marker and label your containers. Better yet, buy a label maker. These lovely printed labels will make your heart sing. Labels can be white or transparent and there are a range of ink colours available. I defy you not to love them!

If I have to write labels, I always go for a black marker and use upper-case letters. I want my labels to last, be uniform throughout the home and clearly legible.

Kitchen labels
As there could be quite a few containers in the kitchen, you don't need to label every single one. For example, if you have a shelf or two with containers of party items such as napkins, candles, plastic cups, plates and fun decorations, simply label the shelf or the drawer. All the containers hold the same category of items, so it's sufficient to have the shelf or drawer as the guide. You don't want your labels looking cluttered.

Toy labels The aim is to encourage kids to tidy up by themselves as much as possible. Once you have organised the toys as you would like them, it is essential that the storage you are using for the toys is labelled. Make it easy for children to know where to find their toys and where everything goes at tidy-up time by labelling as soon as possible.

Labels can be written but I find a photo label is best. Not only are they nicer on your storage because they're as bright and colourful as the toys themselves, but kids, especially younger ones who haven't learned to read yet, can see much more quickly exactly where each toy is supposed to go.

Take nice photos of some Lego, a train set, figurines, crafts, etc. Or simple clip art can be printed, coloured in and added to storage. Fix the image on the front of the storage bin you are using and voila! Or, for older children, use bright Sharpie pens in a variety of colours to write the labels.

Shoe labels One of the most beautiful labels you can create. Your shoes aren't organised until you have a photo on the outside of the storage. If you keep your shoes in their original boxes or in clear shoe boxes, having a small photo on the outside not only allows you to easily recognise what's inside, it also looks gorgeous. Absolute perfection in every possible way – design, decor and function.

Bedroom labels Minimal labelling is needed in a bedroom and wardrobe, but the labelling you can do can be fabulous. Containers in the less accessible upper wardrobe shelves would benefit from labelling. Labels for memorabilia, photos, travel items, etc. will look well and clearly indicate what is located in these hard-to-reach areas.

Any containers that have a handle on them can have attached labels with twine, which look cute wrapped around the handle. Tags usually reserved for your gift wrap can be used to re-create this look.

For cloth storage, try using a pen that writes on material.

When you are storing items long term, clear labels on the outside are essential to jog your memory. For example, if you have a box of clothes and inside there are some seasonal and some baby clothes, you would write that on the box, for example 'Summer clothes – adult' and 'Baby clothes – memorabilia'. You could add an inventory list inside the box, for example:

- Clare's summer clothes

- John's hiking gear

- Oliver's baby clothes 0–3 months

- Oliver's baby clothes 4–6 months

If you have multiple boxes for a single category, label the boxes as per the example below. For instance, you have a few boxes for ski gear, which you've labelled 'Ski gear'. If you have more than one box, you would label them 'Ski gear – Box 1 of 2', 'Ski gear – Box 2 of 2', etc. Then add an inventory list specifying what's in each box.

BOX 1/2 CLOTHES	BOX 2/2 ACCESSORIES
Jackets	Goggles
Trousers	Masks
Gloves	Sunglasses
Scarves	Helmets

Finally, when you put bags or boxes in the attic, always mark the date. Boxes and bags can spend years in the attic before you get to look at them again, never mind declutter. By marking the date on the outside every time you deal with the bag or the box, you will clearly see the last time you sorted it.

These labels add a rustic French charm or Hamptons beach vibe to your storage. Chalkboard labels can be stickers or attached with twine. Use chalk or a chalkboard marker to write on them, and simply wipe *clean if you need to change the label. They're perfect for kitchens and laundry rooms.*

Office labels *The office needs a lot of labels. It's a working environment, so a more serious label style works very well here. Label as much as possible without making it look cluttered.*

It's essential to label paperwork. Keep to black and white, and use capital letters to maintain uniformity throughout the room. More details on labelling paper are in Chapter 17.

Labels that wrap around wires are very cute and will help you identify which wire belongs to which plug for each piece of equipment without having to unplug them.

USING THE METHOD

Over the following chapters, we will start putting the method described in this chapter into practice in the rooms in a home. You will see that the bathroom, living room, attic and garage spaces are not in this book. The rooms chosen are the main rooms I have been asked to organise by my clients over the last number of years. Makeup and toiletries, the main items found in the bathroom, are instead covered in the bedroom chapter. Similarly, sometimes the living room is part of an open plan area that encompasses the kitchen and toy room, so you may find that instructions in Chapters 10 and 14 would work for the living room too. The method explained can be used in any room and any space.

When you tackle any room, there is preparation before and clear-up afterwards. As we've seen in this chapter, there are three steps in each stage.

	PREPARATION	TASK	CLEAR UP
1	Gather your supplies	Categorise	Tidy up
2	Set a time limit	Declutter	Storage
3	Tidy up	Organise	Labelling

As we move on to the room chapters, I will outline the most important steps of categorising, decluttering and organising that make up the *task* of organising. I will also discuss storage. The other steps that constitute *preparation* and *clear-up* should be done every time you organise, but to avoid cluttering up these pages – and your head – they won't be repeated.

Now that we've got that bit of housekeeping out of the way, are you ready to get organised?

One of the most common questions I'm asked is *'Where do I start?'* My advice is to begin with a flat surface. So let's do just that.

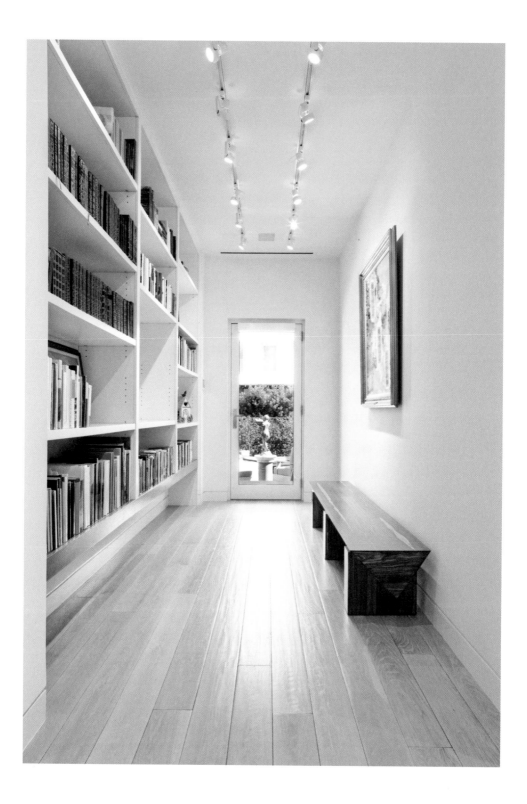

9

FLAT SURFACES

·

FLAT SURFACES CAN BE KITCHEN AND BATHROOM COUNTERS, KITCHEN ISLANDS, DESKS, BEDSIDE LOCKERS, MANTELPIECES, WINDOWSILLS, COFFEE TABLES, TV UNITS OR BOOKSHELVES.

·

The largest flat surface is the floor. Cluttered surfaces, including the floor, can be very oppressive. They're guilt and stress inducers. One client described looking at her surfaces covered in paper as '*visual noise*'.

·

If you clear a surface, you will immediately feel better. You won't even realise how much clutter is affecting you subconsciously until you remove it. All of a sudden you can breathe. My clients feel this relief and they are unsure why, until I point out that we cleared a surface.

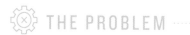 ## THE PROBLEM

Flat surfaces are magnets for clutter. They're the equivalent of junk drawers, but at least with a drawer you're not looking at it all the time. They work the same way, however; they're full of random bits and pieces that you have to rifle through – usually under pressure – in the hope of finding what you're looking for.

Common surface problems are:

- Too many surfaces in the one room

- Large expansive surfaces that attract a lot of clutter

- Seen as easy solutions for whatever is in your hand

- They facilitate procrastination

- They are a constant reminder of tasks to do

- Items to be put away are left out for days

- There is a mix of miscellaneous items

- Piles of paper gather

- They lead to embarrassment when visitors arrive

- They are always a mess, need constant tidying

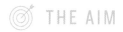

The aim is to clear your direct eye line, which will allow you to think clearly, and give the illusion of more space because the area directly in front of you is clear. This will give you a good start to your tidying and decluttering and ensure you feel more comfortable and more in control of your space and your stuff.

On your journey to becoming more organised, focusing on keeping surfaces clear is the number one lesson. 'Clear' sometimes means devoid of everything. More often it merely means clear of things that aren't supposed to be there.

 BEFORE YOU BEGIN

As your largest flat surface, the floor is an entity all of its own. If clutter builds up so much that you are starting to lose floor space, it's time to do something about it. Whether it's paper piled on the floor, one too many items kept 'just in case', or too many pieces of furniture, if there's more clutter than carpet, something has to give.

For rooms that are simply full of too much stuff, don't immediately think of decluttering them, just tidy them. Move items on the floor right over into the corners of the room, keeping one corner with nothing in it. You need to have some floor space to give you room to manoeuvre, let the space breathe, and help improve the flow and feel of the room.

When that's done, you can get into the nitty gritty of what's on the floor by following the walls. Take one wall at a time and declutter using the method described later in this chapter. As you move around the room, the cluttered sides will start to reduce and the side containing items you need to keep increases. The items to keep are then moved, once the cabinets, drawers and units in the room are clear.

Too much furniture can be a real obstacle to the organisation of a room. If you have furniture that you've been meaning to get rid of, now is the time to do so.

Perhaps you had some bedside lockers in your master bedroom a few years ago. Following some redecoration, one locker is now on the landing and the other is in the guest room. Perhaps you could get rid of the one on the landing.

A living room containing a mix of modern furniture and furniture inherited from family members may need some consideration. Sometimes removing just one piece is all it takes to give the room a little breathing space and physical room to manoeuvre, thereby enhancing the ability to get it organised.

An organised space does not have to mean a minimal space, with everything decorated in a pale colour palette and with no decor. Spaces can be full of vibrant colours and different patterns yet look beautifully organised and uncluttered. There are various factors that contribute to that, but the most important factor is a clear floor space.

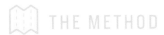 THE METHOD

Let's look at the flat surface hot spots again.

- Kitchen islands

- Kitchen counters

- Mantelpieces

- Windowsills

- Bedside lockers

- Tables

- Desks

- Chests of drawers

- Empty or almost empty shelves

❶ CATEGORISE

In the living room, remove the clutter from the windowsill and mantelpiece and place the items on a clear table or clear piece of the floor.

In a bedroom, remove the clutter from the bedside lockers and spread the items on the bed.

In an open plan living/kitchen area, gather up the clutter from any surface (counters, islands, units, shelves) and place the items together on the table.

Examine exactly what tends to land on the surfaces regularly. It is usually the same suspects time and time again.

- IN THE LIVING ROOM, there may be candles, essential oils, party accessories, memorabilia, old Christmas cards, wires and cables, pens.

- IN THE BEDROOM, there are probably magazines, newspapers, books, toiletries, makeup, wires and cables, medicines, Lego.

- IN AN OPEN-PLAN LIVING/KITCHEN AREA there might be school work, arts and crafts, shopping, keys and wallets, stationery, receipts, laundry.

- ON A DESK, you'd probably find paperwork, pens, stationery, receipts.

❷ DECLUTTER

Taking each category, go through one by one and reduce what you own. Remember your four decluttering bags. Throw rubbish out to general waste and recycling. Create a pile for items that belong elsewhere and distribute at the end. Create another pile for items to be donated or returned to family and friends.

Don't allow rubbish accumulate on your surfaces. Throw it out as soon as you can. Leaving it out makes everything seem worse than it actually is. In actuality you're not looking at clutter to be dealt with, you're looking at rubbish that could have easily been thrown out days ago!

❸ ORGANISE

In order to figure out how you are going to organise these items, stop the spread and create a long-term system, you need to question what the items are and why do they end up on your surfaces?

SCENARIO 1	SCENARIO 2	SCENARIO 3	SCENARIO 4
They simply land here because you haven't had time or you're too tired to put them away, e.g. a morning of shopping has resulted in bags being left on the kitchen table.	Items need to be left out because they are relevant, e.g. a note for school that your daughter forgot to take with her this morning, a doctor's appointment card, a broken ornament that needs gluing, a gift for an upcoming birthday.	Items have no home, e.g. stationery, arts and crafts, schoolwork.	Items simply belong in the bin, e.g. random receipts, loose plastic, unused manuals.

All these situations result from habit and lack of time. It seems easier to mindlessly leave things on surfaces 'to get back to' later than to sort them out now. Your perception that you either don't have time, or that the task would take too long, has created a habit that continually leads to the same result – clutter on your surfaces.

ACCEPT GOOD ENOUGH

In a busy household, it may be rare to have surfaces that are clear, but there are ways to limit the number of surfaces that are falling prey to clutter. For example, you enjoy arts and crafts with your kids and need to leave the supplies and creations out overnight, so you usually place these on a surface – the kitchen island, a table or perhaps a cabinet surface. The next morning you open the post and you leave out some bills you need to pay. Later, your sister calls round with some clothes she thinks you might like to borrow and they have been left draped across the dining room table.

With a lack of time, remember to consolidate. If you must clutter a surface, clutter only one! Keep all random items on one surface only. Yes, it's still out, but that's the point: you can still see it, so you're reminded that you need to do something with it. Confine it, but get back to it, okay? This will help keep the rest of the room tidy. Just tidying clutter onto one surface only, even without actually organising and decluttering anything, can make you feel better. The space appears tidier and you can actually use it. Better yet, when you do this simple tidy-up, you will inevitably end up putting one or two items away, so you've made a start.

WITH A LACK OF
TIME, REMEMBER
TO CONSOLIDATE.
IF YOU MUST
CLUTTER A
SURFACE,
CLUTTER ONLY
ONE!

STOP CREATING RANDOM BOXES

Many people, when they're in a hurry, shove items into the spare room, into a cupboard or into a random box or plastic bag. Please do not do this. I have decluttered many a random box. 'Tidying' items away like this allows you to close the door on the clutter – literally and figuratively – for weeks on end. Eventually you can't remember what's in the bag in the corner of the room or dread to look at what's in the spare room.

SHOPPING ITEMS

Shopping items are a no-brainer; they should go straight to the room where they belong. If you've bought a new black dress, but you've no room in your wardrobe, it doesn't matter. The dress does not belong on the kitchen table and that's for sure. Don't delay putting things in the room where they belong just because that room isn't properly organised.

TO-DOS

There will always be to-dos around the home. If any of these to-dos can be done in less than two minutes, do them. For instance, the school calendar you've been meaning to stick on the wall. Do it now. The shoelaces you've been meaning to change. Do it now.

If you need to leave items out to remind you to do something, keep them consolidated together as described above. Noticeboards, for paper reminders, or shallow baskets on surfaces are handy to keep items like these together. It stops the spread and when you need them you have only one place to look. Ideally, by improving your time management, you won't have to leave them out as reminders. Your to-do list and schedule will do the reminding for you.

SCHOOL SUPPLIES

With school supplies in the kitchen, is there an area near the kitchen island where you could create a small nook? Having a dedicated space, even a small one, will make it quicker and easier to put these items away. Or try a portable option. Get a nice basket for school items, for instance, and place items in here when it comes time to tidy up. Pen holders on the desk or kitchen counter, or dividers inside shallow drawers, corral stationery together. Check out ideas on zones in Chapter 8.

PAPERWORK

Paperwork organisation is described as part of creating a household management folder in Chapter 8 and again in Chapter 17.

Your habits around what you do with the item in your hand, plus your habits around time, must change in order to stop items continually landing on surfaces. As we saw in the beginning of this book, it all comes full circle back to you!

Mastering flat surfaces will prove very beneficial to you and the organisation in your home. It can speed up your tidying and gives you a good start for your larger decluttering projects too. To get the home organised and keep it organised, remember to keep your flat surfaces clear.

There's a surface in every room, so keeping that learning in the back of your mind, let's move on to specific rooms in the home.

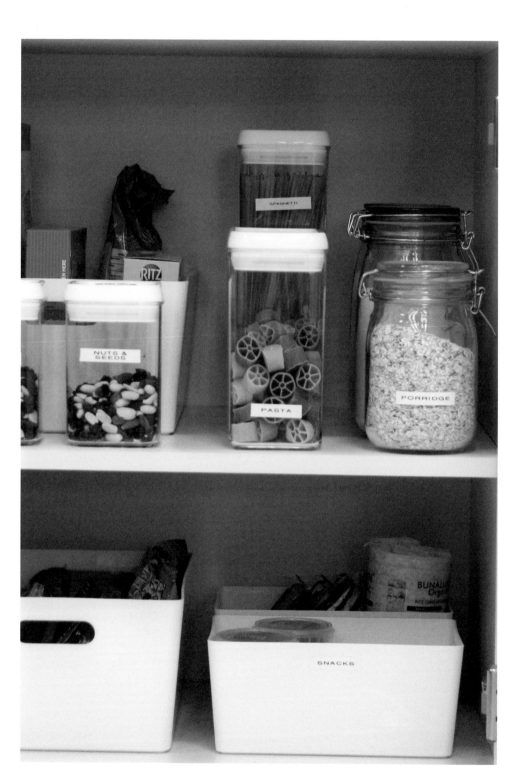

10

KITCHENS

·

LET'S PAUSE FOR A COLLECTIVE SIGH!

·

The kitchen is the high-traffic area of the home. People are in and out all day long, bringing with them an array of items. It's a never-ending love story between clutter and counter top – they're drawn to each other like magnets – and you're left looking on despairingly. You know it won't end well, and you'll have a right mess to clear up soon. Why can't clutter just fall in love with the bin instead and leave you out of it?

The kitchen environment is made up of ecosystems that you find elsewhere in the home. You have the wardrobe in the form of the pile of laundry growing in the corner; the office is the stationery and paperwork that huddle on the counter; the hallway is the school bags, jackets and shoes that are torn off and 'homed' on the floor; there's even the garden shed, with hardware, small gardening tools and seed packets making their presence felt in the junk drawer.

THE PROBLEM

- Too small.

- Too big.

- Too much food – you buy extra because you can't find what you have, and some is out of date.

- Deep, dark presses or cabinets too high.

- If you bake a lot you need a lot of supplies, many of them very small, which can be difficult to home in a standard-sized kitchen.

- The kids' school work, arts and crafts are scattered around the kitchen.

- Manuals for various appliances around the house are in a muddle around the kitchen.

- Paperwork for the house, or brought home from the office, the Sunday newspapers and reminders on Post-it notes gather on multiple surfaces.

- The island is never clear and always gathering clutter.

THE AIM

To create a hub in the home that allows life to flow. A space that caters for eating, learning and creativity. A warm space that is easy and functional and nurtures family life. A room to welcome unexpected guests or hold a party.

It can be difficult to get a kitchen organised if you don't do it in one fell swoop. As there are so many cupboards, drawers and presses, starting in one place will affect the next. It's best to dedicate at least a morning to the kitchen so that you can complete this task all at once rather than dipping in and out of it.

❶ CATEGORISE

Take a step back and examine the presses and cupboards as they currently stand. Usually there will be a few areas that don't need any work. For example, your cutlery drawer probably doesn't need to be touched. Under your sink may need to be tidied but in general it works well. Take note of these areas as space that is not available to you.

Now look at the cupboards that are available to you. They are full and cluttered right now, but these are the ones you will work on, create space in and re-home items in a system that makes sense.

Not all kitchen decluttering and organisation requires changing everything around. In fact, it's rare that this happens. Often, emptying a few presses gives you enough room to manoeuvre in order to create organisation across all the cupboards.

First, start to categorise. Pick a cupboard or cabinet and empty it completely to create your blank canvas. Now sort through the items you removed. Use a kitchen table or island to spread items out. Imagine the kitchen table as a grid. Different categories will be placed in different squares of this imaginary grid. For example, put all the pots and pans in the top right-hand corner of the table. In the next imaginary square, you place all baking equipment, in the next imaginary square you place all food.

Continue creating categories as you move throughout the kitchen. If your table or island gets full, use the floor. Keep the categories separated and neat so that you don't undo all your work.

Here are a few examples of categories and an inventory of items in each that can be found in an organised kitchen.

TABLE DRESSING	COOKING	BAKING	FOOD
Crockery	Pots and pans	Baking trays	Fridge
Glasses	Steamers	Cake pans	Vegetables
Cups	Juicers	Mixing bowls	Confectionery
Cutlery	Pressure cooker	Weighing scales	Dry foods
Napkins	Deep fat fryer	Mixers	Canned food
Tablecloths		Blenders	Cereals
Candles			Baking goods
			Spices and herbs
			Sauces, oils
			Jams, spreads

PACKAGING	CLEANING PRODUCTS	HEALTH	FAMILY ADMINISTRATION
Aluminium foil	Bin bags	Medicines	Paperwork
Clingfilm	Wipes, polishes	Supplements	School supplies
Sandwich bags	Disinfectants	First aid supplies	Stationery
Baking paper	Paper towels		Daily post
	Washing up liquid		
	Laundry products		

❷ DECLUTTER

By now you will have categories similar to those in the table. Some of these categories will be spread out on your kitchen table, counters or floor; others may be still in the cupboards and drawers.

Taking each category, go through and cut through what you own. You need to make space now.

Decluttering is most effective when done by category. If you are looking through serving dishes and bowls, make sure all your serving dishes and bowls are together. When you keep together like with like, it's easier to decide what stays and what goes. You have a bird's eye view of everything, not just bits and pieces.

Sort through medicines and food by their use-by dates. Check pots, pans and cooking utensils. Unless you're a chef, you don't need ten ladles, five sieves and nine bread knives. Remove discoloured, mismatched or broken crockery and Tupperware.

❸ ORGANISE

Now that we know what we're keeping and in what categories, it's time to put everything back. But in a much more organised way!

Always match the size of the categories you need to home with the size of available space.

CABINETS

In the food category, the tallest items are usually boxes of cereal. Therefore, you will need a tall cabinet or shelf for the cereal. Putting the cereal box in a tall cabinet answers our question about food storage. We want to keep the food category all together to form a zone, so all other non-refrigerated food will go in the cabinets and shelves around the cereal. Tall shelves are also good for storing spaghetti (if you keep it standing upright), and they should also be used for large baking trays. Remember, the bulkiest, tallest, most used item always gets priority of space. Then everything else falls in around it.

DRAWERS

Shallow drawers hold food preparation items such as tinfoil, clingfilm, sandwich bags. They also hold folded towels and aprons, napkins, candles and tablecloths.

Deep drawers or the back of deep presses are best for bulky kitchen equipment and for items that are least used, such as glassware, crystal, tea sets and vases.

KITCHEN ISLANDS

Kitchen islands and tables can be the ultimate clutter hotspot. You eat here, work here, do school homework here, so the array of items that land on these areas can be vast.

The first thing to realise is that the island will need tidying every day if you don't want clutter building up. When something lands on an island, it is very visual. If that drives you crazy, you need to either tidy it once a day or get rid of the island. Drastic, but as we've seen, large furniture sometimes needs to go.

To keep clutter to a minimum here and to make tidying it easier, remember that it's a flat surface, so you need to examine what exactly tends to land here regularly and put solutions in place to catch these things.

COUNTER TOPS

I always keep one section of counter completely clear. This is between my cooker and my sink. When I prepare meals, it's much easier to have this clear space to work.

Aside from the impracticality, having something on every inch of counter can be quite claustrophobic. Keeping one segment totally clear will lift the entire kitchen. Decide which segment can remain free of content. It doesn't have to be a large space; it could be a small area of counter space behind the door. Having some parts of the countertop free is not only more aesthetically pleasing, it also gives you space to actually use your counters. If you have a small kitchen, you may think that you can't achieve this, but you can!

Group together the items you need on the counter: usually the kettle, toaster, maybe a fruit bowl and bread bin. Ensuring that there is a socket, place the kettle, toaster and bread bin together first. You have now created a small zone that will be very efficient at breakfast time.

UNDER THE SINK

Place the cleaning and laundry supplies you use most often in this space first. If you have duplicates, overflow or excess stock of these items, they can be left here if space allows; otherwise, try creating a 'kitchen zone' in your laundry/utility room.

In order to avoid cross-contamination, keep sponges and cloths for the bathroom separate from those used in the rest of the house. In this area, you might also have some sponges for outdoors or for pets. Colour-coding sponges for each type of use and labelling them will keep everything separate, organised and healthy.

ABOVE THE CUPBOARDS

Don't forget the tops of the cupboards. If you have multiple items in the far reaches of the kitchen, they can look dirty and disorganised. Give these upper areas a good clean to remove dust and grime. Ideally, your kitchen will be organised enough that you can keep this area clear. However, if your cabinets are full, you may have to resort to using the space above them. This isn't ideal, but there are ways to make this neat and organised-looking.

Only use the space above one or two cabinets; don't spread things out over the tops of every cabinet because this will make the room feel claustrophobic – the exact opposite to what you're trying to achieve. Try using the tops of corner cabinets, so that the items will appear more 'tucked away'.

And finally, assign only items that aren't used very often here. Items such as vases or large serving dishes work well in these spots – they can even look quite pretty.

CORNER UNITS

These tricky areas can be difficult to organise. Their awkward shape can restrict what you can put in and they're usually quite deep and dark. These units are best for items that you don't use very often. Large kitchen appliances that aren't needed every day are ideal in these spots, and stocks of medicines, DIY supplies and drinks also work well here. If the corner units are next to your oven, use them for pots, pans and dishes.

When placing items inside, place them in order of use. For a two-shelved corner unit, imagine it is divided into four – bottom shelf back, bottom shelf front, top shelf back, top shelf front. The bottom shelf is less visible and less accessible than the top. The back of the bottom shelf is least visible; the front of the upper shelf is most visible.

Place items inside with this in mind. The closer you come to the front of the upper shelf, the more frequent the items' use.

Remember access. You must make sure that if you are placing items in front of one another, as will often happen, you only ever want to have to move one object to get to something behind it. You don't have to fill every available inch of space. If there's not much in the corner units, pull the items towards the front so they're easier to get at and leave the deep space behind empty.

JUNK DRAWERS

Every home has a junk drawer (or three). Very often, the items found in these drawers can also be found in smaller piles throughout the kitchen too. Mismatched items huddle on small shelves, have fallen behind a row of cookery books or are having a party on your windowsill.

This is usually where I start in a kitchen. It's important to note that none of these items is junk. They are all important and needed. They also all belong together but can be organised in a much more efficient way so that they are actually used. To tackle these items, you have to take an aerial view.

Here are some items that regularly fall into the 'junk' category:

- Light bulbs
- Batteries
- Screwdriver/ hammer
- Plant/vegetable seeds
- Pens, pencils
- Post-it notes
- Paperclips
- Rubber bands
- Photographs (loose)
- Passport photographs

- Receipts
- Sunglasses
- Sunglasses cases
- Old medication
- Herbal remedies
- Napkins, straws, cake candles
- Candles, nightlights
- Cigarette lighters, matches

When organising the junk drawer, the first thing to do is toss the contents out on a kitchen or dining room table or kitchen island. Then categorise the contents. But how do you categorise them and where do you home these items so that they don't end up back in a junk drawer and will actually be used? Let's take the items above and look at some suggestions for where you can sensibly re-home them.

ITEM	NEW HOME
LIGHT BULBS	Laundry/utility room/under the stairs/upper kitchen press
BATTERIES	Laundry/utility room/under the stairs/upper kitchen press
SCREWDRIVER/HAMMER	Shed/garage/laundry/utility room
PLANT/VEGETABLE SEEDS	Shed/garage/laundry/utility room
PENS, PENCILS	Home office/kitchen counter/kitchen drawer
POST-IT NOTES	Home office/kitchen counter/kitchen drawer
PAPERCLIPS	Home office/kitchen counter/kitchen drawer
RUBBER BANDS	Home office/kitchen counter/kitchen drawer
PHOTOGRAPHS	Home office/living room/upper shelves of a wardrobe/attic
RECEIPTS	Home office/kitchen drawer
SUNGLASSES AND CASES	Bedroom/car/handbag
OLD MEDICATION	Throw out
HERBAL REMEDIES	Kitchen press
NAPKINS, STRAWS, CAKE CANDLES	Kitchen press
CANDLES, NIGHTLIGHTS	Kitchen press/living room
CIGARETTE LIGHTERS, MATCHES	Kitchen press/living room

These items are literally everywhere in a kitchen and very often they are found in pockets throughout the rest of the home too. Lightbulbs and batteries are under the stairs, sunglasses are in the car, medicines are in the bathroom.

So it takes time to filter through these items and decide, once and for all, where exactly you want them to live. Remember, *you are setting the item up for its next use.* Always ask yourself, next time I need this item, where would I look for it? Where would I be? What would I be doing? That leads you to the potential home.

While you are looking at these items, think if you have seen the same items in other places around the home. For example, you might have medicines in the bathroom upstairs. On decluttering the kitchen you have found medicines here too – in fact more here than upstairs. You have a few options now:

1   THE MEDICINES UPSTAIRS ARE BROUGHT DOWN TO THE KITCHEN AND THEY ALL LIVE HERE.

2   THE MEDICINES FROM THE KITCHEN ARE BROUGHT UPSTAIRS AND THEY ALL LIVE IN THE BATHROOM.

3   THE ADULTS' MEDICINES ARE KEPT IN THE KITCHEN AND THE KIDS' MEDICINES GO UP TO THE BATHROOM (YOU DON'T WANT TO HAVE TO COME DOWNSTAIRS IN THE MIDDLE OF THE NIGHT IF THEY'RE SICK).

4   OR PERHAPS YOU COULD SPLIT UP THE MEDICINES INTO THREE: ADULTS' IN THE KITCHEN, KIDS' IN THE BATHROOM AND FIRST AID IN THE UTILITY ROOM.

Again, asking yourself, 'What would I be doing when I need this?' can help you determine the best home.

❹ STORAGE

- CONTAINERS: I like to use white or clear containers so that items are clearly visible. Uniformity helps the organisation. Also get containers that are easy to wipe clean.

- MAGAZINE FILES: These are excellent for stacking baking trays. When they're stacked they're easier to access and don't fall over.

- LAZY SUSAN: Because this item spins, it's useful in a deep, awkward space.

- S HOOKS: One of the handiest items in a kitchen. They allow you to hang multiple items from a variety of unusual spots, from rails to door handles.

- CABINET DOOR HOOKS: For hanging towels, dustpan and brush.

- SLIDING OPTIONS: Baskets that slide in and out on a runner can make a huge difference in the kitchen, making the back of dark presses or very high shelves more accessible.

- **WICKER BASKETS:** Get the French country decor feel in your kitchen. They are lovely for a variety of items, from vegetables to cookery books to day-to-day paperwork.

- **BISCUIT AND CAKE TINS:** Give cakes, chocolate, biscuits or sweets some nice storage instead of leaving them loose. If you have some that you don't want the children to access, get two; one for healthy snacks, one for treats.

- **DRAWER DIVIDERS:** If you must have a junk drawer, have a tidy junk drawer. Measure inside the drawer and get dividers to fit. Keep items from sunglasses to a measuring tape and pens neatly corralled inside the dividers.

And finally, a word about lighting. For deep, dark alcoves, add sensor strip lights that come on as you open the press door. Or add a battery-operated push light. Good lighting is essential for helping to maintain the organisation of a space.

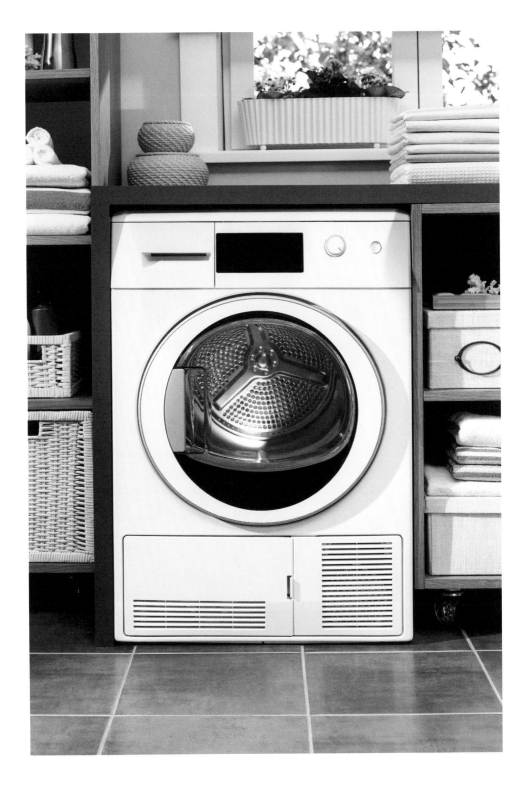

II

LAUNDRY ROOMS

·

IN A BUSY HOUSEHOLD, LAUNDRY CAN SEEM AS IF IT GOES ON FOR DAYS.

·

In almost every home I visit, one of the biggest
complaints is how to organise
the laundry, either the room itself or
the routine around it.

·

Utility and laundry rooms can hold a large array of items. Of course, they contain the essentials for cleaning and drying the family's clothes, but they often act as an extension to the kitchen, garden shed and bathroom.

There are often a lot of stock items here too. Spare toilet rolls, cleaning products, even wine. Stock is all well and good, and it's a very organised notion – provided there's the space for it. If not, the space gets cluttered, the stock can't be found or accessed when needed and duplicates, or even triplicates, are purchased.

Common problems here are:

- You can't find anything because items cross over with items in other spaces.
- Space is too small.
- Space is too large.
- Abandoned hobby materials.
- Too many shoes.
- Too many coats.
- Several people use the space, including (perhaps) the cleaner.
- Never-ending clothes mountain.

◎ THE AIM

A clean and clear space facilitates a constant flow of clothing and constant family member access, maintains cleanliness and avoids cross-contamination. If you have a cleaner, a clear laundry room will facilitate his or her work.

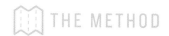

Laundry/utility rooms or spaces are usually quite small and happily can be organised in a very short period of time. So let's go!

❶ CATEGORISE

Work around the room. Start with the floor, then move on to the counters, then any shelving, drawers or cupboards. Pick up everything and place each item into categories. If the room is very small, you'll have to pull items out into the nearest room to spread out. Most utility/laundry rooms are an Aladdin's cave.

Categories to be considered include:

LAUNDRY	CLOTHING	SPORTS GEAR	OUTDOOR/ DIY	EVERYDAY ITEMS	KITCHEN STOCK
Dirty clothes for washing	Shoes	Sports clothes	Tools/DIY equipment	Handbags	Medicines, first aid equipment
Clean clothes for ironing	Summer/ winter accessories	Sports equipment	Outdoor gear	School bags	
Ironed clothes to be moved to bedrooms	Coats, jackets	Tennis balls, golf balls, rugby balls, footballs			Stock of food
Towels					Extra vases and other kitchen items
Bed linen					
Irons, drying rails and baskets					

Not to mention the large items: washing machine, tumble dryer, ironing boards, sweeping brushes, mop, vacuum cleaner, microwaves and sewing machines. And they all need a home.

As you move around the room, categories will build up. If you find items that do not belong, place them in a separate 'belongs elsewhere' pile.

❷ DECLUTTER

Now go through each category and remove anything you no longer want or need or that is broken or damaged.

LAUNDRY

Declutterer beware: towels and bed linen can take longer than you expect. Allow for that. Create your sets and go through one by one to see what you need to keep. Sets without matches can be kept as spares for accidents, guests or second homes. Donations of bed linen and towels are not always welcome, so check in advance with the charity of your choice.

Worn, discoloured, stained and generally old towelling and bed linen can be thrown out.

Take note of new sets you may need and keep that in mind when allocating space in your organising stage.

Irons, microwaves, sewing machines, drying rails, baskets are awkward, bulky and take up valuable space. Do you really need two microwaves or three irons? Put aside for electrical disposal. Make sure rails and baskets aren't broken and can be used as intended.

CLOTHING

Shoes in this room can be examined as part of the larger shoe collection when working in the bedrooms. If there aren't too many shoes and a quick declutter is possible, go for it. Remove any that are too old or worn. Remove any shoes that are not supposed to be here for redistribution to the bedrooms later.

Winter/summer accessories are sometimes particularly difficult to find. A lone swimming armband will often be floating in the laundry without its mate for months on end until it's finally tracked down in the shed. As with shoes, declutter what you can now. Remove anything too small for the children, anything without its match that you wouldn't want even if you had the match, anything stained or simply too old. Throw out sun lotion over a year old, swimming aids that are no longer needed now that the kids can swim, and straw hats that are out of shape.

If you have coats and jackets here it's usually because your laundry room is near the back door. If they're here now, then I'm guessing they will stay and we will create a zone for them.

With that in mind, remove any coats or jackets that you don't want or that don't fit any more. If you are splitting coats and jackets with space elsewhere – for example a bedroom – put coats for that area to one side. If there are coats in that other area and you'd rather they were here, bring them to this space.

SPORTS GEAR

Any items in this category that are in this space are usually for hobbies or after-school activities. Items that don't fall into these categories should be moved to outdoor storage if you have it.

These items can be awkward, so only keep what you really need. Do you really need six hockey sticks? Will you ever get round to restringing that tennis racket? Do the kids play with all five footballs?

Keep all the paraphernalia together: not just clothes, but supplies too, such as bicycle lights, pumps, locks, etc. Each hobby will get its own basket or drawer later.

OUTDOOR/DIY

Unless you are an avid gardener or DIY enthusiast, it can be difficult to identify some items in this category, let alone know whether you should keep them.

Don't worry about being able to identify nuts and bolts, screws and rawl plugs. All those little items can be simply grouped together. If someone in your life can identify them and their use and is happy to declutter them, great. If not, keep them together and move on to a more difficult category. Don't waste time decluttering a group of items that won't make much difference to the overall organisation of the space anyway.

On the other hand, if you are a gardening or DIY fan, we need to honour your hobby and source of joy. If you love it, why is it such a cluttered mess? Perhaps you find that you don't get a chance to garden or flex your DIY muscles as much as you like? Maybe that's because you can't find your supplies. Look after the things that make you feel good. You are the expert here. Declutter anything you know you're not going to use.

Finally, get rid of any unnecessary multiples, items covered in rust, anything broken.

Wellington boots, rain gear, fluorescent jackets, buckets and spades, tents, picnic items, rugs and mats all fall under the category of outdoor gear.

Separate out by person if you wish, or keep everything all together. It depends on how much you have in this category. The more you have, the more you may need to sub-divide.

Items such as tents and foot pumps are very bulky and if you have any outdoor space, it's essential for your indoor space that those items are moved out. If your children are getting older, how likely are picnics any more?

Check sizes, permeability, wear and tear to help you determine what stays and what goes.

EVERYDAY ITEMS

The only handbags, school bags and sports bags that should be here are the ones currently in use for work and school, and they should get priority spacing, whether on hooks on the wall or shelves. This room is busy enough without multiple forms of baggage.

If, after you have completed the organisation of the room, there is space for other bags, you can add them then. But deal with the priority bags first.

KITCHEN STOCK

It's not unusual to have a mini extension of the kitchen in the utility/laundry area. Go through all items in this category and make sure they are all in date and in use. Categories are dealt with in the same way as with the decluttering and organisation of the kitchen.

The only kitchen items in this space are those used least often. The most used items get priority spacing in the kitchen. Items here are excess or stock. The organisation of any kitchen items in this room should reflect the organisation currently in your kitchen.

❸ ORGANISE

In order to design where each item will go, you have to know what items are priority for you in this space. For example, if your laundry room is near the front door, you might prioritise sports supplies and school bags so that the minute the kids walk in the door, they have somewhere easy to dump their stuff in an organised way. If it's close to the kitchen, you might prioritise space for stocks of food, and space for sports gear will be a little further back.

Think about how you want to use this space and how you want your family to use this space.

Keep the items that are used most often on shelves, in drawers and in presses that are easiest to access. And remember: match item size with available space.

COUNTER SPACE

To keep a laundry routine working and avoid backlogs, good counter space (or designated floor space if you have no counter) and good baskets are essential to keep clothes moving through the cleaning stages. Creating space for laundry baskets coming into and out of the room must be prioritised.

CABINETS AND SHELVING

Supplies such as washing powder, dryer sheets, etc. should be placed on the shelves or in the cabinets located closest to the equipment. They are top priority and given prime placement.

After that, categories as below can be assigned to cabinets and shelves, bearing these guidelines in mind.

Coats, hats, scarves, gloves, sunglasses, Wellington boots, shoes, rain gear, tissues, etc. are located closest to the door that leads outside. If there is no door to the outside, and the laundry opens into the kitchen, these items should be close to the kitchen so that you don't have to venture too far into the laundry room to find them.

If you have a garage or outdoor shed, items for gardening, DIY, tools, etc. need to be out there. Keep a measuring tape and a hammer if you wish, but all other items in this category need to be zoned outside.

If you don't have a garage or any outdoor storage at all, dedicate a shelf or upper cabinet space and put everything you need for the garden and home maintenance there.

Extra kitchen supplies should be placed nearest the kitchen.

WALLS AND BEHIND DOORS

Use the walls and behind the doors to the max.

Drying rails, ironing boards, sweeping brushes and mops can all be hung up along a wall. But don't hang items on every square inch of wall space as this will make the room look cluttered. Have at least one wall that is just that; blank wall space.

Look behind the cabinet doors. Can you hang anything relatively flat, such as cloths, or perhaps a dustpan and brush?

DRAWERS AND PULL-OUT BASKETS

Assign sports supplies, small equipment and clothing to drawers and pull-out baskets. Give each drawer its own sport. For example, in a three-drawer system, one could be cycling, another swimming, another dance.

Alternatively, you could assign a drawer to each family member, for example the top drawer is for the eldest and it contains all his tennis gear; the middle drawer for the middle child contains all her ballet gear; and the bottom drawer for your husband's cycling supplies.

DEEP DRAWERS AND HIGH SHELVES

Buckets, spades, picnic items, rugs, etc. are compact and rarely used so can be assigned a deep drawer or a wide top shelf and neatly put away.

❹ STORAGE

Laundry rooms can be the perfect balance between function and beauty. With some good design you can make your laundry room luxurious. Imagine, luxury in a laundry room!

EQUIPMENT

Storing washing and drying machines on top of one another instead of side by side can save space.

LAUNDRY BASKETS

It's great when laundry baskets fit inside cabinets or on their own shelves and you can pull them out. If you have tall space under a counter, assign three cabinets (dirty clothes, dry clothes, ironed clothes). Each cabinet contains a basket for each stage of the routine.

HANGING RAILS

A hanging rail between cabinets for recently ironed clothes looks gorgeous.

HOOKS

For walls and behind doors, hooks are your go-to solution. They can be used for coats if you store them here. However, if there is any way you can put up a rail, I would opt for this. It will be much neater, easier to use and less visually unappealing if it gets messy. Rain gear and fluorescent jackets can be included with coats and jackets, or you might prefer to fold them and add them to your sports category. Shopping bags can have a hook at the back of a door. School bags can be assigned a hook, placed low down for each child.

SHOE SOLUTIONS

If you have shoes in this room, spend time thinking through how you will organise them. Shoes kept here are usually used every day. If there are kids running in and out of this room, pulling on runners or firing dirty football boots back into the room, you want something that's going to catch all this activity. Shoe rails are usually not great in this room because the rails aren't strong enough to withstand the constant grabbing of shoes. Sturdy shelves may work better. For kids' shoes, baskets might work best. They can stand at the laundry room door and throw shoes in from a distance to their hearts' content, but at least the basket looks pretty and the huddle of shoes inside doesn't disturb the rest of the room's organisation. Pick your battles! Trays with pebbles inside can look pretty for Wellington boots or hiking boots but are most practical in a minimalist laundry room.

MASON JARS

Glass jars can hold pegs or night lights, or you can even decant washing powder into them. This is really making a display of your storage.

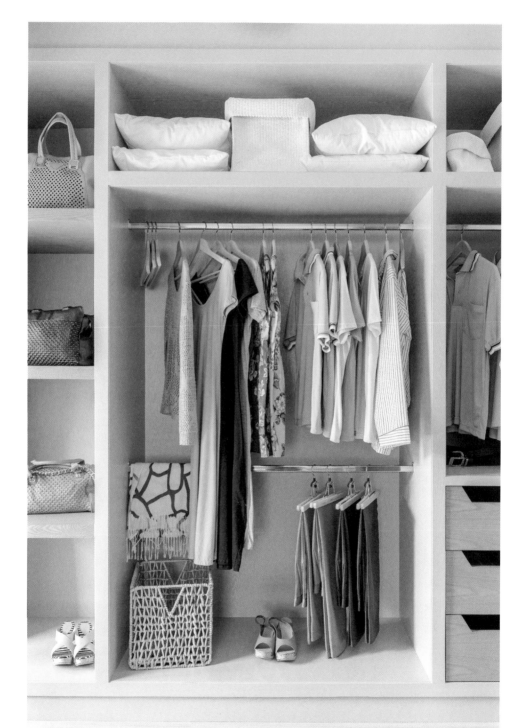

12

WARDROBES

·

WARDROBES CAN BE A VERY EMOTIONALLY CHARGED SPACE TO ORGANISE BECAUSE OUR WARDROBE HOLDS THE ARMOUR THAT WE FACE THE WORLD WITH.

·

Clothes are very important to some people;
less so to others. Either way, our clothing gives us
a sense of identity. They can make us feel good
or feel awful.

·

If your clothes aren't making you feel good and you also have the uncomfortable feelings a disorganised wardrobe can cause, well, your wellbeing can take a hit.

THE PROBLEM

- Too many clothes.

- Lack of storage.

- Enough storage but too full.

- Broken door frames, handles, shelves, drawers, hangers.

- Unsure where to start and how.

- Wearing the same outfit multiple times a week.

- Wearing the clothes at the front of the wardrobe, on the floor or on the bedroom chair.

- Resorting to wearing black.

- Nothing clean or ironed when you really need it.

- Constant build-up of laundry.

- Multiple wardrobes and you're unsure what's in each.

- Your clothes are in the wardrobes in your children's bedrooms.

- Sharing the wardrobe with uneven distribution of space – partner has no room.

- Wardrobe full of miscellaneous items, from children's toys to Christmas decorations.

THE AIM

There are so many reasons why having an organised wardrobe is a must!

You wake up in the morning and there's not a garment in sight. You open the wardrobe doors and enjoy the ease as it swings open and doesn't jar. You know exactly what you're going to wear. Or you may have the luxury of pondering what's on the rail. There's no thought involved. Everything is there and if it's not you know it's only in the laundry. Garments are neat, accessible and fun to pick out and wear.

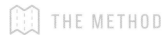 ## THE METHOD ···

There are enough problems in life already – opening the wardrobe and choosing an outfit shouldn't be one of them. So if it is, let's fix that, shall we?

❶ CATEGORISE

As you take clothes out of the wardrobe, spread the categories out on the bed. Imagine the bed divided up as a grid, and each box in the imaginary grid is assigned a category of clothing.

How would you like to categorise? For example, you examine a black pair of jeans. Ask yourself, when I go to look for my black pair of jeans on Saturday night, where will I want to find them?

I   **WILL THEY BE AMONG ALL MY OTHER JEANS?**

2   **WILL THEY BE WITH ALL MY OTHER EVENING WEAR?**

3   **WILL THEY BE WITH THE CREAM LACE TOP I ALWAYS WEAR WITH THEM?**

How you think determines how you sort and categorise your clothing. For example, your answer might be one of the following:

I   **YES, AMONG ALL MY JEANS.** Therefore you put the black jeans into your one 'jeans' category.

2   **SOME JEANS WILL BE WITH MY EVENING WEAR, SOME WILL BE CASUAL.** So you add the black jeans to your 'evening' category.

3   **YES, I LIKE TO CREATE OUTFITS.** So you add the black jeans to your cream lace top, put them both on one hanger, and create the outfit. You then combine all your outfits onto the rail.

Once you settle on how you're going to sort, follow that system as you move through your clothes.

In this section, I'll follow the system of organising clothes by type, so I'll categorise it under type of garment. I'm not going by outfit or how I would wear it.

On one side of the bed, you will put your winter clothes and on the other your summer clothes. Each season will then be divided into a category. Very often an item of clothing is worn all year long – it's neither winter nor summer – especially in Ireland. I find it's best to prioritise winter clothing, as generally that clothing works all year round. If you do not wish to divide your clothes by season, you can ignore this step.

The inventory of items we would expect to see in the categories that make up your wardrobe are as follows:

CLOTHES	HANDBAGS	SHOES	ACCESSORIES
Suits	Day bags	Everyday shoes	Belts
Blazers	Evening bags	High heels	Ties
Trousers	Beach bags	Runners	Hats
Jeans	Clutches	Flats	Scarves
Dresses	Wallets	Ankle boots	Pashminas
Skirts		Knee-high boots	Gloves
Shirts			Wedding accessories
Blouses			
T-shirts			
Sweaters			
Tracksuits			
Swimwear			
Holiday clothes			
Underwear			

Let's get started. Work each section of the wardrobe – rail, drawers, cubby holes, lower shelves, upper shelves.

CLOTHES

Take each item off the rail, touch it, feel it and look at it. You have to take the hanger out and really look at it. If you flick through the clothes on the rail, you may find one or two pieces to get rid of, but most will stay. But if you take the hanger off the rail and out, and really look at it in the light, you will make a better decision on each piece.

Taking a blouse off the rail, ask yourself, 'Is it a winter blouse or summer blouse?' Add it to the 'blouse pile' for the relevant season on the bed. Continue with each piece of clothing as you move along the rail. The piles of clothing, separated on the bed, continue to grow. Remember to imagine the bed as a grid with each category of clothing assigned an imaginary square.

Then move on to any drawers and shelves that hold clothes. Pull all the clothes out, put them on the floor and sort from there. This gives you a blank canvas to work when you come to organise and it forces you to look through every piece of clothing. Again, examine each piece of clothing and add each type of clothing to the corresponding pile.

Your clothes may be spread over more than one wardrobe. For example, you may be creating a 'work wear' category in your master wardrobe, but you know there are also work suits in the spare room wardrobe. If that's the case, go to the spare room wardrobe and pull out your work wear. Do not pull anything else out and do not get distracted. Do not start working on that wardrobe. Go in, get the category of clothing you need and get out!

And the same thing applies vice versa. If, when organising your master wardrobe, you find one or two pieces of golf gear there, but most of it is in the spare room wardrobe, then take the golf gear from the master wardrobe and move it to the spare room. Again, don't worry if that wardrobe is a mess. Just put that category of clothing in it and get back to the main event. You will get to the next wardrobe in time. For now, you are categorising and only focusing on the clothes you want in the master wardrobe.

Remember, if you are looking at skirts, look at *all* your skirts. If you're looking at trousers, look at *all* your trousers.

HANDBAGS AND SHOES

Bring all your handbags and shoes together. They may all be in your bedroom, but usually they're also in the hall, utility room or even the car! Do you want one large category or do you want to split these? Do you want all handbags in one place and all shoes in one place? Or are you happy to split them? For example, you might want all evening bags and shoes in the master wardrobe, and all sports bags and shoes under the stairs.

Gather all your accessories together to create this category and to see clearly how much you own. Do not include jewellery yet. Jewellery will be dealt with in the next chapter.

❷ DECLUTTER

Before we begin, there are a few things to think about.

SENTIMENTAL ATTACHMENT

There's a lot of sentimental attachment to clothing out there. As I help people sort through their clothes, almost every item has a story associated with it. The dress, the top, the cardigan is a reminder of a person or an event in their life. Old baby clothes can be particularly difficult for parents to let go. Keeping some clothes for sentimental reasons is okay, within reason! And if there are items you deem too important to toss out, put them in the attic or at the top of a closet and don't let these clothes take up the space that clothes you need today require.

GUILT

Many of us keep clothes that we hope to wear again one day. However, I'm not sure it's a great idea to have a lot of clothes in your wardrobe that remind you of a size you used to be and hope to be again. As they hang there, they are a constant reminder that you are no longer that size. And this can bring on a feeling of guilt, and you begin to associate the wardrobe and clothes with feelings of inadequacy.

Whatever about keeping one or two items, as we all do, anything more takes up space in our heads, never mind our wardrobe. And as for those one or two items, I wouldn't keep them in direct eye line either.

Guilt can also appear when we start to look at all the money that was spent on clothes that are now lying in bags ready to be thrown out or donated. A lot of people make decisions to keep items of clothing just because they feel that they will get their money's worth if they do. But it's hardly getting your money's worth if they never leave the wardrobe. In fact, if you send them to a charity, someone else will get good use from your old clothes, and *that* extends the life of the clothing and by extension its monetary worth.

Deciding what clothes to keep or throw out can be as painful as walking home in high heels after a night out.

Keep these questions in mind as you forage through your fashion.

I   WHEN DID I WEAR IT LAST? IF YOU CAN'T REMEMBER, IT'S BEEN TOO LONG!

2   DO I REALLY THINK IT WILL COME BACK INTO FASHION? AND IF IT DOES, WILL I STILL WANT IT?

3   IF I WERE OUT SHOPPING RIGHT NOW, WOULD I BUY IT AGAIN?

4   IS IT WORTH THE SPACE IT'S TAKING UP IN MY WARDROBE?

5   DOES IT FIT? IF NOT, IS THE GOAL TO FIT BACK INTO IT ACHIEVABLE AND MOTIVATING?

6   HOW MANY OF THIS TYPE OF ITEM DO I HAVE AND DO I NEED THEM ALL?

7   IS THE ONLY REASON I'M KEEPING IT BECAUSE OF HOW MUCH IT COST?

8   DO I REALLY HAVE THE TIME AND ENERGY TO GET THIS ITEM REPAIRED?

9   DO I REALLY HAVE THE TIME AND ENERGY TO SELL THIS ITEM?

10 HOW DOES THIS ITEM MAKE ME FEEL?

II   DO I EVEN LIKE THIS ITEM?

CREATING YOUR 'MAYBE' PILE

Don't waste time humming and hawing over clothes you're unsure about. Create a 'maybe' pile and keep going with the other items. At the end, come back to these 'maybe' items. Your subconscious will have had a chance to catch up and hopefully will make your decisions easier.

Do not keep these clothes because you're too tired or because space has opened up. You need to keep the clothes because you really love them or need them; not because you're fed up. It would be better for you to leave these 'maybe' clothes out until you're sure one way or the other. If you do that, give yourself a deadline for your final decision, otherwise the clothes will remain.

Okay, here we go. You have looked through the clothes and categorised them in a way that works well for your habits. Now it's time to take each pile and reduce what you own.

CLOTHES

As you're going through your clothes you will find items that need to go into the laundry, taken to the dry cleaners or sent to get altered. Your immediate reaction will be to throw them in the wash or create separate piles for the dry cleaners, etc.

Please don't do this. You may feel uncomfortable putting dirty or damaged clothes back in the wardrobe, but to analyse space effectively you need to. What if you get to the end of your wardrobe organisation and all the space is taken up? What will you do when the dry cleaning comes back or the washing is done? You have to assign *all* your clothes to *all* your available space.

Co-ordinate the organisation of your clothes with the end of a laundry cycle. Do your decluttering when you have very little or no laundry to do.

For items that need to be dry cleaned or fixed, make note of them, finish the organising and then you can go back and take out these items for the errand at hand.

Try the clothes on if you need to. It will make the organising process that little bit longer, but it might make the decision of what to keep and what to throw out that bit easier. However, do keep an eye on time. You will get less decluttering done, but your decluttering will be more precise.

HANDBAGS AND SHOES

These can be very difficult to declutter. People love their handbags and shoes, they are often an investment and some women have quite a lot of both of these types of item.

Selling items like these takes an investment of time. There are consignment shops that will take your items and sell them for you, which I think is the best use of your time. Create a separate pile of handbags to be sold as you go through them.

If you struggle to let these items go, start by getting rid of the shoes and bags that are very old, dusty and worn, which should stand out and be easier to let go. That will create a bit of a dent in your collection (I hope!).

Keep the questions above in mind as you go. Remember, you love these items. They are a collection and should be treated as such. Therefore poor-quality, worn, old shoes and bags need to go so that we can create a beautiful display and highlight this love and the hard work it took to earn these items. Keep that in mind. Identify the ones you really really love and get rid of the ones that don't serve you any more. If you create some space, you'll be able to indulge your love of them and buy another. Think of it as a reward for all these difficult decisions!

And remember to empty out your handbags, whether or not you're keeping them.

ACCESSORIES

Scarves are usually the biggest group of accessories. From winter to evening, silk to summer, there are drawers stuffed with scarves in our wardrobes. Even with our weather, we can all manage to declutter a scarf or two. Continue to reduce ties, hats, belts and other accessories that make up this category. Get rid of flattened sun hats, frayed ties and belts that belonged to your '80's wardrobe.

NO-BRAINERS

The following items should be thrown out without a second thought.

1 ANY CLOTHING THAT IS DAMAGED AND CAN'T BE REPAIRED

2 ANY CLOTHING THAT IS STAINED OR DISCOLOURED AND CAN'T BE CLEANED

3 ANYTHING WITHOUT ITS MATCH – SHOES, SOCKS, GLOVES, ETC.

4 OLD TIGHTS, POP SOCKS AND UNDERWEAR

OTHER ITEMS TO GO

Items such as children's toys, books, CDs, stationery, etc. do not belong in your wardrobe. Take them out and if you are not throwing them away, re-home them. The only things that should be in your wardrobe are things you wear.

FROM NOW ON

Consider placing a donation bag at the bottom of your wardrobe. This can be a plastic or paper bag, a small laundry bin; whatever is convenient for you and the space in your wardrobe. Over the next while, any clothing you come across that you don't want or like, or can't fit into any more, and that you would like to donate, toss it into this bin. When it's full, take it straight out for donation and replace the bag with a new empty one.

❸ ORGANISE

Now we have a bed full of clothes, but at least we know they're clothes you actually want. You have a pile of clothes for donation and a few rubbish bags too. You also have your blank canvases to work with – an empty rail and empty shelves. Now we'll organise and give every category of clothing a specific section of the wardrobe. Make sure to polish the shelves and hoover the base of the wardrobe before putting anything back in.

IF YOU HAVE MORE THAN ONE WARDROBE

If you either have too much to fit in one wardrobe, or you simply like the idea of separating out your belongings, make sure you use each wardrobe for a different category of clothing. Each wardrobe has a different job to do. For example, the wardrobe in your bedroom is for the clothes you use most often. Wardrobes in other rooms could contain all your coats, or your evening dresses, or your (or your partner's) golf and hiking gear. For example:

WARDROBE 1	WARDROBE 2	WARDROBE 3
WORK CLOTHES:	**ALL OTHER CLOTHES:**	Coats and jackets
Dresses	Tops	
Shirts	T-shirts	
Suits	Lounge and sports wear	
	Trousers	
	Blouses, etc.	

IF YOU HAVE A WALK-IN WARDROBE

There are usually multiple rails in a walk-in wardrobe, and each rail should hold a different category of clothing. For instance, gym gear on one rail, dresses on another, suits on another, tops, shirts and blouses on another. The same principle applies to drawers and shelves. For example, all pyjamas in one drawer, all underwear in another, all scarves in another, etc.

If you have some sports gear hanging up and some folded in a drawer, make sure that the rail closest to this drawer is the rail for sports gear. If you have clothes for work hanging up, but some work tops folded, the rail you designate for work wear should be nearest to the drawer holding work clothes. Always keep the zones as close together as possible.

On the shelves, put all handbags, wallets and clutches together, all perfume together, all jewellery together. Items in the same category should be in the same area.

If you need to use high shelves for your clothes, use them for clothes that are sturdy. Higher shelves mean you have to stretch. When you stretch and pull you're more likely to topple clothing and create a mess. So choose folded jeans or folded skirts; these will hold their own if pulled and are easier to keep organised.

If you need to put T-shirts, vests and other flimsy clothing on a high shelf, put them in a drawer divider or basket first and then up onto the shelf.

Suitcases that need to be homed in your wardrobe go on the upper shelves. If they jut out, try tucking them on the floor of the wardrobe instead. If you travel regularly, have your suitcase(s) within easy reach.

The upper wardrobe shelves are the perfect spot for a box or two dedicated to memorabilia and sentimental items. They can also accommodate handbags well.

Make sure to hang up awkward clothing such as blouses and cardigans. Blouses can be very flimsy and difficult to fold and keep folded, as can cardigans.

As you place clothes on the hangers, dress the hanger as you dress yourself. Fix the top button of the shirt, close the zip on the jacket, tie the ribbon at the back of the maxi dress.

Keep clothes facing the same direction. The front of the garment should be looking into the back of the next garment, all facing the same way.

Keep categories together. If you have categorised by type of garment, then keep all dresses together, all shirts together, etc. If you have categorised by activity, keep all work clothes together, all casual clothes together, etc.

Each cubby hole or shelf gets a category of clothing. When you were categorising, you will have separated T-shirts, sweatshirts, string vests, evening tops, so now assign a different category of clothing to each cubby hole or shelf, giving them a 'job' to do.

Cubby holes can also be a good space for handbags, and the lowest cubby holes on the floor of the wardrobe are good for some shoes, e.g. slippers, flip-flops, sandals.

If your wardrobe has drawers, smaller drawers are assigned smaller items – socks, lingerie, silk pyjamas, scarves, winter and summer accessories.

Large, deep drawers are assigned bulky items – jeans, sweatshirts, sweaters, tracksuits.

Drawers that are broken need to be fixed immediately. It'll affect all your organisation if you don't. If you can't fix them, try to avoid using them.

The wardrobe floor is good for shoes. If you decide to put shoes elsewhere and/or there isn't enough space on the upper shelves for suitcases, the suitcases can go here.

Where do you want to keep your shoes? Do you want all of them near your front door, or all of them in your bedroom? Do you want some in both areas? If so, be specific about which shoes are homed where. Two areas max would be my recommendation. Otherwise you're back to square one, with too many homes.

Make sure that whatever item you choose to locate here does not hit off the clothes hanging from the rail above. Clothes that drape over a large suitcase, or cover shoes, lead to clutter. If the clothes hanging from the rail sweep to the floor of the wardrobe, avoid using that area for storage completely.

❹ STORAGE

Now that we have put everything back into the wardrobe, let's make it even more gorgeous with some storage solutions.

- SLIMLINE, FELT HANGERS are essential for every wardrobe. They allow you to maximise available rail space and they hold your clothes on the hanger very well. You won't have blouses or cardigans falling off the hangers.

- WOODEN HANGERS are excellent for suits, coats and jackets. If you have enough space on your wardrobe rail you could forego the felt hangers and go for all wooden. However, there are certain garments that will only stay put on a felt hanger.

Matching your hangers is guaranteed to bring the organisation in your wardrobe to another level. However, if you are on a tight budget, there are ways of matching hangers without completely overhauling your stock of hangers. If you have a mixture of plastic, wooden and felt hangers, you can group those along the rail. For example, assign all your wooden hangers to your coats and put them all together on the rail. Give all the plastic hangers to your dresses and place them together. And so on.

This uniformity will make the wardrobe look better. When the same type of hangers are all together they work better together. They are all the same shape and size, so they fit in with one another. This creates sturdiness on your rail and helps reduce the chance of garments becoming messy.

- RAIL DIVIDERS are slotted onto the rail of your wardrobe and labelled. They divide the rail by the clothes categories you create. If the wardrobe is arranged by clothing type – dresses, suits, blazers, shirts, etc. – or by season, activity, etc., the dividers indicate this organisation across the rail. They are excellent for kids or if you share a rail.

- SHELF DIVIDERS help keep your handbags standing up straight. They will also keep jumpers and jeans neatly on shelves and prevent garments falling over.

- CUBBY HOLE CONTAINERS help keep your handbags standing up straight. They will also keep jumpers and jeans neatly on shelves and prevent garments falling over While tops, jeans and jumpers can be folded inside cubby holes, having items such as hair supplies, toiletries and jewellery loose on these shelves will only look messy. Get baskets or other containers that fit snugly inside the cubby hole and places loose items inside. One category per cubby hole.

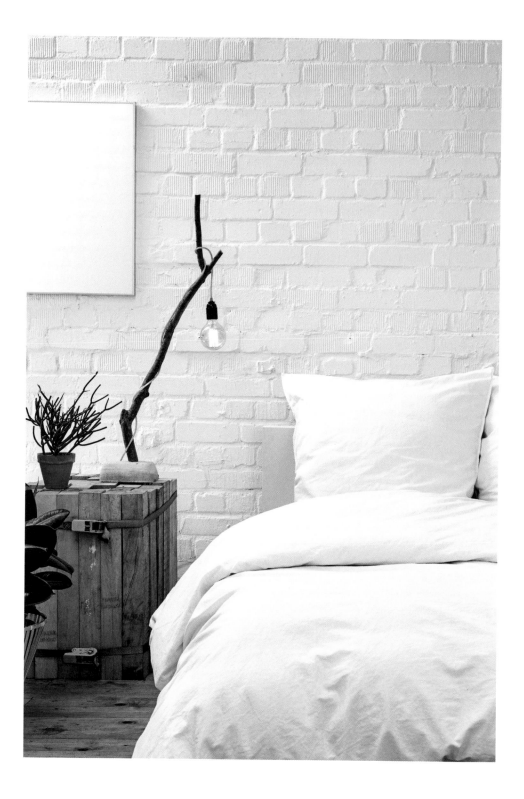

13

BEDROOMS

•

IN MY OPINION, THE BEDROOM IS THE MOST IMPORTANT ROOM IN THE HOUSE.

•

The bedroom is our place to retreat from the world, a very private area. It's your space, containing your things, comforting you when you're sad or sick, facilitating sleep to help you grow, nurturing your most precious relationships. *This is the space where you can be at your most vulnerable.* The real you is here. Every aspect of your physical, mental and emotional wellbeing is looked after in this space.

•

Not only do I think it's important to keep these rooms free of clutter, I think it's a responsibility. You are responsible for looking after your health and wellbeing. You can't take care of others if you don't take care of yourself. If you're neglecting your bedroom, I believe you're neglecting your health and the essence of you.

A space that holds such strong emotions and has the power to influence how our day starts and ends needs to work for us and not against us.

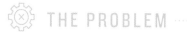 ## THE PROBLEM

Waking up in a room that you don't like starts your day on a pretty bad note. The day hasn't even begun and you're frustrated. And it's the same every evening. When you go into your bedroom, you recoil, and that's not a feeling associated with good rest and recuperation. Remember, it's not good to go to bed angry.

- Too much furniture or furniture too big for the space.

- Lack of storage.

- Decor that is old and neglected.

- Areas in need of repair and renovation.

- Too cold.

- Too much stuff.

- Items from other areas of the home.

- Acting as storage space for non-bedroom items (e.g. Christmas decorations).

- Unfinished jobs – a headboard that should have been sold, picture frames that were never hung.

- Sharing the space with young children for too long.

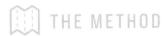

THE AIM

A sanctuary to relax in and enjoy. A place where you can sleep and rest, where you care for your family and relationships, where you enjoy your most personal things that you have worked hard to own. Whether you are running in and out of the bedroom to grab shoes, or you only have five minutes to throw on a tracksuit, you want to be able to do so without any hassle and without thinking.

THE METHOD

We have just looked at clothes and items that help you dress – shoes, bags, accessories. Now, we'll deal with everything else that can accumulate in a bedroom.

❶ CATEGORISE

Below are some sample categories found in a bedroom. Taking each section of the room, start gathering items into their categories. Non-clothing categories that are typically found in a bedroom include:

- Makeup and toiletries: foundation, eye shadow, lipstick, mascara, primer, bronzer, tanning products, nail polishes and remover, creams for face, body, hands and feet, shampoo and conditioner, hair colour, soaps, samples

- Jewellery and perfumes: perfumes, perfume samples, necklaces, bracelets, rings and earrings, watches

- Office and paperwork

- Books

- Personal interest

- Hair supplies: brushes, combs, bobbins, hair clips

- Kids' stuff: baby toiletries, clothes, toys, blankets and cloths

❷ DECLUTTER

Each of the categories can be quite big, so you may wish to take one at a time instead of doing everything in one go.

MAKEUP AND TOILETRIES

You may find that organising these items takes longer than you anticipated – this is a huge category. You have been warned! You will have more toiletries and makeup than you realised, and going through these things takes time. Reduce what you own by whether you have allergies to any items, whether they are out of fashion or out of date, etc. Use-by dates on makeup are represented by a symbol of an opened tub. The opened tub has a number such as six or twelve on it, suggesting that the makeup should be thrown out six or twelve months after opening.

JEWELLERY AND PERFUMES

Jewellery is a category that can be tackled on its own. If you can declutter it in 20–30 minutes, then by all means do so. However, cluttered jewellery can take quite a while when it is old and knotted. You don't want to spend so much time on jewellery that the rest of the room doesn't get done. In that instance, it's best to bring all jewellery together in one place in the bedroom, get on with the rest of the room, and then one evening as you're watching TV you can take care of the jewellery as a separate project.

Perfumes and aftershaves, on the other hand, are an easy category that should be quick to declutter. No excuses!

OFFICE AND PAPERWORK

Give paper its marching orders. Banish it for ever from this room. It can go wherever you want, just not in the bedroom. The only exception to this is if you are in a tiny home or apartment and you must have an office area in the bedroom. In that case, declutter it to its bare bones. Scan and digitally store as much paper as possible.

As you work on the bedroom, group all the paperwork together into a pile but unless it's a very small amount, don't spend time sorting through it. We'll deal with decluttering paperwork in detail later.

BOOKS

Peter Walsh, the American organising guru, suggests that *for every 10 books you get rid of one*. However, even this is too difficult for some. Where do you want your books? In an ideal world, where in your home would you like them? One spot is best, but, as with shoes, you may like some in the bedroom, and the rest somewhere else. As you declutter the books, separate out the ones you are keeping into 'bedroom' and 'elsewhere'. Leave the 'elsewhere' pile of books at the door for distribution later.

PERSONAL INTEREST

Old ticket stubs, lanyards, fridge magnets, posters, diaries, etc. are items that are special to you and yet don't belong anywhere. The only thing they have in common is that they spark a memory for you. I often find these items scattered throughout a wardrobe or bedroom with no proper home. These very special items are treated in a not so special way. As you go through the room and, in fact, your entire house, you will find many of these items. Getting a system set up for them now will give you a landing spot for all the others you are bound to find along the way.

BEDROOM FURNITURE

Less is more when it comes to bedroom furniture.

Having a chair in the bedroom can be a lovely addition to the room. However, they are a huge clutter magnet and if you find that the chair is more often a mess than used for relaxation, it might be time to remove this clutter magnet! Chairs should only be in bedrooms if you have the space and you don't mind actively keeping them clear.

If you have lockers either side of the bed that aren't being used, don't open properly, or prevent drawers in the bed being opened, perhaps floating shelves might be a better idea.

Are there any other large pieces of furniture in your room that you're not using and could go somewhere else or be given away? Losing worn-out furniture will lighten and brighten the bedroom.

❸ ORGANISE

Let's look at the available space typically found in a bedroom, what may be homed there, and the zones we can create. *Match category size with available space.*

BEDSIDE LOCKERS

Items such as our diary, pens, our current books, magazines, medicines, music, candles, aromatherapy, writing supplies, etc. are of personal interest to us. They help us relax, learn, grow. So the best zone for these types of item is one that's close to us, such as a bedside locker or a nearby chest of drawers. Items that work well in bedside lockers are:

- ✓ PERSONAL INTEREST
- ✓ BOOKS
- ✓ TOILETRIES
- ✓ MAGAZINES
- ✓ EMERGENCY SUPPLIES/MEDICINES
- ✓ TORCH
- ✓ DAY-TO-DAY JEWELLERY
- ✓ SPECTACLES

UNDER THE BED

This space is good for any of the following categories:

- ✓ UNDERWEAR – ALONG WITH DRAWER DIVIDERS TO KEEP IT ORGANISED
- ✓ HANDBAGS
- ✓ CHUNKY KNITS
- ✓ PYJAMAS
- ✓ SPORTS WEAR AND TRACKSUITS

✓ **SHOES**

✓ **MEMORABILIA**

✓ **PHOTOGRAPHS AND PHOTO FRAMES**

BOOKSHELVES

If you have books, CDs and DVDs in your bedroom, chances are you have them on a shelf of some sort, and this home makes perfect sense, so there's no need to change it. Don't make this process harder on yourself by changing what works.

I'm not a huge fan of books in the bedroom. Certainly having some books in the bedroom is good for relaxation, but too many can be claustrophobic. If you are stuck for space, I would prioritise items that you need for getting dressed over too many books.

Bear in mind that bookshelves can be used for non-book items too, e.g.:

✓ **SHOES – THEY CAN LOOK FABULOUS LINED UP**

✓ **A LINE OF PRETTY WICKER BASKETS CONTAINING TOILETRIES, MAKEUP, JEWELLERY**

✓ **A DISPLAY OF PERFUMES**

SURFACES

The surfaces in your bedroom will make or break its serenity. Items placed on surfaces should be homed there with purpose. The items designated for surfaces should hold their own. Smaller, loose items can be on these surfaces but held neatly together in storage.

Remember, when you walk into your room, your subconscious registers the surfaces first. So don't put anything on them you don't want to see in your new, peaceful bedroom.

CHEST OF DRAWERS SURFACE

Probably the largest surface in a bedroom, it can be a useful space for storage, just don't overfill it. Think of the rule of threes - something to the left corner, something in the middle and something to the right corner.

- ✓ DISPLAY TRAY CONTAINING YOUR PERFUMES

- ✓ DISPLAY TRAY FOR YOUR AND/OR YOUR PARTNER'S WATCH, LOOSE CHANGE, ETC.

- ✓ JEWELLERY BOXES

- ✓ TISSUE BOX

- ✓ SOME BOOKS WITH LOVELY BOOK ENDS EITHER SIDE

- ✓ ALARM CLOCK/CD PLAYER/SOUND SYSTEM

- ✓ TWO TO THREE OPEN CONTAINERS OR BASKETS LINED UP THE WIDTH OF THE UNIT CAN LOOK GOOD. INSIDE PLACE MAKEUP, TOILETRIES, LARGE COSTUME JEWELLERY, SUPPLIES FOR A BABY

BEDSIDE LOCKER SURFACE

The top of the locker has a very specific job to do. It holds everything you need to hand for relaxation. No toys, paper, work documents, technology, etc.

- ✓ ONE OR TWO BOOKS

- ✓ A COASTER

- ✓ TISSUE BOX

- ✓ PEN AND NOTEPAD

- ✓ SMALL CONTAINER FOR THAT DAY'S JEWELLERY

WINDOWSILLS

Please, please keep them clear. For me? No? Okay, if you can't, stick to larger items. Small items loose on a windowsill scream clutter – even if you know exactly what's there and use everything. If there are small items needed on this surface, get a nice open basket and keep them all together.

- ✓ SOME BOOKS

- ✓ A FEW ORNAMENTS

- ✓ A SELECTION OF PHOTO FRAMES

Books, paperwork and equipment should be in the bedroom as a last resort only. However, if you use your bedroom as an office, mark out a clear 'office' zone. If you have a desk, make full use of the space above and below it. Use the entire length of the wall, adding shelving. Keep paperwork inside box files and other storage so that you don't have to look at it. Invest in pretty storage and nice labels and make a feature out of the office space. If you have to look at work-related paraphernalia, at least make it look uniform, calming and inspiring.

CRIBS OR CHANGING TABLES

If you're sharing your room with your children, a clear zone to separate their things from your stuff will help keep everything organised, and also help preserve your sense of self.

If you have a crib or changing unit in the room, keep supplies for the kids in a zone beside this furniture. Use the space above and below these units as much as possible.

❹ STORAGE

On your mission to create your oasis of calm, organisation will be streamlined through lovely bedroom storage. Because the bedroom is used every day, add the storage in as quickly as you can to maintain the organisation you've now put in place.

DRAWER DIVIDERS

These are very important in any bedroom. Placed inside chests of drawers, bedside locker drawers, under beds, even deep cubby holes, they keep like with like in an organised fashion. It's easy to see what's inside and easy to pull items out and put them back again.

Dividers allow you to zone the inside of drawers or along shelves. Categories are held within the divider and then the divider creates the zone. For example, in one single bed drawer, you could have drawer dividers in one half of the drawer containing your underwear and then on the other side of the drawer is your nightwear. There is a clear division.

Certain drawer dividers come divided into sections of nine or twelve and that storage is great for belts, scarves, socks and tights.

OPEN BASKETS

Once again, they add a rustic feel to your bedroom. They can be used on the surface of your chest of drawers or the upper shelves of a wardrobe. Use them for items such as hair supplies, scarves, winter accessories, empty toiletry and makeup bags.

UNDER BED

If you have bed drawers, drawer dividers as described above are essential to keep garments together and organised.

If you don't have bed drawers, large cloth containers with a handle or shallow containers on wheels mimic the idea of a bed drawer. They allow ease of access and good storage. Use this solution for shoes, handbags, memorabilia, travel items, out-of-season clothing.

JEWELLERY STORAGE

There are a variety of ways to store jewellery in a bedroom.

Using mirrored or display trays can beautifully store large jewellery such as bangles. They are also good for your perfume display.

A standard jewellery box works for smaller pieces of jewellery. They often run out of space, however. Jewellery boxes that come in sections are very useful as you can expand and stack the storage as your jewellery collection grows (which of course you totally have under control now, right?!).

Use a tray or small box on your bedside locker. When you take off your daytime jewellery, you can place it here.

Costume jewellery is particularly difficult to store as it's so bulky. Necklaces can also be difficult as they tangle easily. A hanging organiser works well for these items as the pockets hold everything. I'd recommend hanging it inside a wardrobe, however, as it can get quite visually 'noisy' if it's out on constant display in a bedroom.

If you are designing a wardrobe, consider storing jewellery in shallow drawers. These drawers can be divided and jewellery organised in the different sections. Drawers with jewellery organised inside can look stunning.

SHOE STORAGE

The easiest and prettiest way to store shoes is on a simple bookcase. However, many bedrooms are not able to fit such furniture. Never fear; there are other options.

There are many different shoe boxes, from plastic to acrylic, transparent to opaque. Boxes such as these allow you to stack your shoes neatly in a corner. Add a shoe label to make access even easier.

Shoe cabinets are useful too. You probably won't get as many shoes into the cabinet as you might expect, so do bear that in mind. Also, the shoes can fall over when the drawer is opened, which makes the inside messy. But I wouldn't worry too much about that. If it's storing your shoes, that's the main thing.

For boots, boot inserts are a must. These inserts keep your boots standing up straight and they stop them falling over, getting damaged and causing clutter.

As many people have a lot of shoes, it's usually necessary to mix and match your storage and use several solutions to home them all.

DECORATIVE BOXES

Choose a lovely box or two for each member of the family for all their special memories. They need to be at least able to fit A4 paper inside. Imagine you are placing a large calendar rolled up inside it, for instance, or some of the kids' artwork. That is the size you are aiming for.

STORAGE OTTOMAN

Placing an ottoman at the foot of the bed can be functional and look very well. It creates a small seating area but doesn't attract as much clutter as a chair. It also offers storage that a chair doesn't. Items that are stored well here include shoes, memorabilia and bed linen.

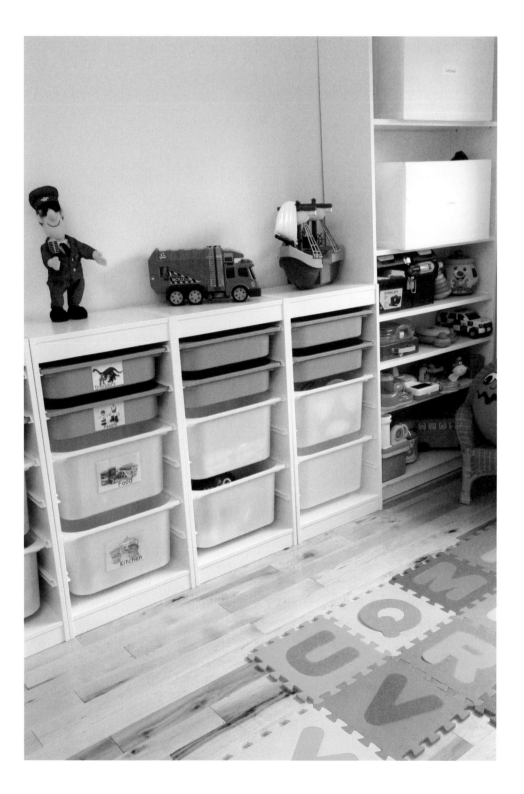

I4

TOY ROOMS

·

OUR LITTLE ONES' TOYS CAN BE SO CUTE BUT THEY CAN ALSO CREATE A NOT-SO-CUTE MESS!

·

We all have too much stuff, but adding a baby into the mix takes what we own to another level. As the kids get bigger, so do the toys, and the smaller our available space becomes. Trying to tidy the kids' stuff throughout the home can seem like a never-ending task. I've met parents who, once the children go to sleep at night and they have time to relax, feel like they're sitting in a playroom rather than their living room.

·

The house is a permanent mess, and there are regular discussions about who's going to tidy up the toys and how. You look into a sea of toys and feel guilty and sad that the kids have so much when others have so little and you're doing nothing about it. All of this causes stress and arguments, and it's a far cry from the fun toys are supposed to bring.

However, it doesn't have to be this way. The key is to declutter regularly and not to over-organise any item they own. Keep items loosely categorised and think about how the kids themselves would look for an item.

THE PROBLEM

- Always a mess.

- Too many toys.

- Not enough storage.

- Not enough homes for the various toys.

- Homes that do exist are too complicated.

- Non-toy items in the toys area – paper, wires, etc.

- Several years' worth of school and art work has been collected and requires sifting through.

- Older kids' things mixed in with toys for young children.

- Kids find tidying up boring.

- Toys are getting lost or broken.

THE AIM

Cutting down on the number of toys, keeping the ones they love or that mean something and having plenty of storage space are the primary goals.

The ultimate aim with organising toys, however, is that the kids will be the ones doing the tidying up. Bearing that goal in mind will help you as you tackle their clutter. It needs to be so easy for them to get at the toys and put them away that it's almost like child's play!

··

To have a toy room or not to have one – that is the question! I wonder if I'll get through this section without dividing the nation.

I have been in many homes with toy rooms and I've spoken to many clients considering dedicating a room to toys. If your decision to have a toy room is simply because there are too many toys all over the house, take a moment and think it through. You may think a toy room will be neater and more organised. That's not necessarily the case. What do you really want to be looking at? What can you live with? What if it's a room that needs regular tidying? Are you okay with that? What would the kids prefer? What might work best to get them to do the tidying? Are there just too many toys?

Whether you have a toy room might depend on how you would like to design the interior of your home and your individual way of organising. Some people don't want any toys in the bedrooms; they want all of them in one room and that's it. One home for everything may be your goal, and a toy room will accommodate that. Ultimately it's your choice. If it's not coming from an avoidance of decluttering, then fire ahead if it's what you'd like to do. The feedback I get from clients is that if you decide to dedicate a room to toys, avoid the front room. The room will often be messy and seeing this mess as you walk into the house will annoy you and it may embarrass you when guests visit. Just a thought from those who have gone before!

From a personal point of view, it wouldn't be for me. First, toy rooms are rarely tidy and I wouldn't want to look at a constant mess, constantly feeling that I need to get round to tidying it, a constant debate with the kids trying to get them to tidy up. Second, even if they are tidy, many toys can be very 'noisy' visually. I wouldn't like a toy room in my main living space. In their bedrooms, the kids can be as messy as they like. I can close the door, it's all contained and out of my direct eye line.

Many of us have outgrown our homes and wouldn't have the luxury of a dedicated toy room anyway. But whatever you do, if you have kids you'll always have toys lying around the house. Whether the toys' 'homes' are the kids' bedrooms or a toy room doesn't matter; you'll still stand on Lego scattered along the hall, you'll still have arts and crafts on the kitchen counters, you'll still find dolls' clothes tucked down the couch. That's kids for you. You can organise their toys to the nth degree, but it really comes down to your attitude: your need for perfectionism; your time; whether you're happy to give time to tidying up; and how you can give the kids more responsibility for their own stuff.

ORGANISING TOYS IN AN EXISTING ROOM

Whether or not you're in the middle of a toy room/bedroom debate, follow the instructions given in Chapter 8 to effectively organise toys in other rooms such as a living room or kitchen area. The aim is to create a lovely play nook for the kids and a clear living space for Mam and Dad to use and relax in.

GETTING THE KIDS INVOLVED

This is like walking a tightrope. You want to get the room decluttered and organised, but should you get the kids involved too? I think it's a great idea to involve the kids, but in a very strategic manner. In my experience, the parent needs to make most of the decisions. You can't declutter large amount of toys or a standard-sized room full of toys and run every toy past your children. It's a nice idea, but you will never get the job done.

Some parents will disagree strongly with me on this, but I'm speaking from experience of both sides of this coin. Generally parents want to check each toy with the kids because they feel guilty about getting rid of their toys. It's completely understandable. But from where I'm standing, which is in the middle of your toy room trying to calm your sense of being overwhelmed, it's your home, your room and your money paid for those toys. It's your time decluttering it and tidying it week in and week out, or your money paying the cleaner to tidy it week in and week out, your money hiring me to organise it. It's your stress levels when you have guests due and the room looks a mess, your pain threshold when you stand on another piece of Lego. It's your time having an argument back and forth over tidying the room or arguing over which toy to keep or get rid of. Is it worth it? Probably not. That all sounds like too much hassle for me, so I come back to the view that you're the parent – and what you say goes. Literally.

If you get rid of some of their toys without them knowing, 90 per cent of the time they won't notice. If they do notice, they get over it. There is a lesson in letting go to be learned here for them.

Let's move on, shall we? Let's think about what to do when the kids are involved.

Most of the kids I have met do let toys go. They know their toys and they know their space because it's all very important to them. However, children like tidiness; they like seeing toys they haven't seen in a while; and most important, they like being asked their opinion. If you ask them where they'd like to home their toys, they usually have a very good idea.

When you are involving the kids, have a strategy. The key is to do the asking and the decluttering quickly. Make sure you're organised and on top of the whole process. They won't be as opposed to doing this work as you think, but they're kids … they'll get bored. So hustle!

Before bringing the kids in, separate out the toys you want them to look at into three categories. One pile of toys that you know must stay. You know these toys, they're important, they're always playing with them, they mean something or they've had them for years.

The next pile is toys you have no connection to at all and you can get rid of them. I wouldn't show those piles to the kids.

The third pile is the toys you'd like to run past the kids; the toys you're unsure about. Get the kids involved in the process. Teach them about decluttering and decisions – letting items stay and letting items go and why.

Finally, be careful that you are not projecting your uncomfortable feelings of letting something go on to your child. They may be perfectly happy to get rid of some things. So when they make the decision, don't make them second-guess themselves. They're learning a great skill in decision-making, and having confidence in their decision will help them with making choices later on. Besides, it might make it easier on you if someone else is making the decision – even if that someone is your four-year-old.

FINDING SMALL PARTS

'I know it's here somewhere!' As you're decluttering, you will find parts that belong to something else, but you can't find that something else! So what do you do with the part? Do you keep it in case it turns up? Do you let it go because you probably won't find the toy, and if you do, you would let the whole toy go anyway? Or are you just not sure?

This happens a lot with jigsaws, board games, wooden toys and educational toys. If you know you won't want the toy even when you find it, then out it goes. If you're unsure, I recommend you have a container or tray for these 'spare parts'. For example, you find a wooden clock; the hands and some numbers are there, but other numbers are missing. Put these loose pieces in a clear bag and place the bag in the container or tray. If you find another piece that belongs to the clock, add it to the bag. If, when you have finished clearing out the entire room, you still haven't found all the pieces – out it goes.

This is a handy method if you plan on donating the item because you can't donate a game or toy with pieces missing. If you deal with loose pieces like this, you can either recycle the toy if it's incomplete or donate a nice toy if you find all the matching pieces.

TOY PACKAGING

No matter the item, I'm a big fan of removing packaging. Not only does the item look better, but you can also get it to fit better into storage.

Removing packaging is not feasible for all toys. For instance, you might want to keep a Lego box because it shows how the toy is to be made or how it fits into existing Lego sets. But with most toys you don't actually need the packaging. In fact, keeping it in the package in order to keep everything together can actually work against you – the pieces still fall out and the packaging looks messy. You could always put toys in a suitable container or a clear bag and throw out the bits of cardboard and plastic.

CHRISTMAS AND BIRTHDAYS

If you do nothing else decluttering-wise, you should at least aim to do some before birthdays and before Christmas. More toys arrive every year, so if you are struggling under the weight of toy clutter already, birthdays and Christmas are the perfect excuse to get some toys out. If getting another influx of toys isn't enough to persuade you to declutter, then you haven't reached your tipping point yet.

Decluttering at these fun, enjoyable and special times can help the kids too. They know they're about to get lovely gifts, so they may be more inclined to let some stuff go. Thinking of others who have less, and being grateful for what we are about to receive, may also encourage them to get rid of things.

If decluttering is done regularly just before these important occasions, it becomes a habit. Everyone gets used to associating a clear-out with certain times of year. Decluttering is helped by routines – and Christmas and birthdays are naturally built-in routines.

Bearing all that in mind, let's get stuck in to what is possibly a very difficult project. It can get complicated and messy pulling out toys on top of toys on a floor, so take your time and create clear boundaries in the room between what is done and what is to do.

❶ CATEGORISE

Your starting point in a toy room are the shelves or cabinets. The aim is to get items up off the floor, so any cabinets or shelving need to be decluttered and organised first.

Taking one shelf or cabinet at a time, take a step back and see if you can see similar toys in it. For instance, you take some Lego from the first shelf. Where else is there Lego? Take all the Lego off the shelves and put it together on the floor. You've now created the Lego category.

Use the same method for everything. If you're looking at toy animals, for example, search for all toy animals. You are now decluttering by category. These categories are building your inventory and will help with homes later.

Once you have categorised all the toys on the shelves or in the cabinets, look at the toys on the floor. Chances are there are several boxes full of random toys there. Turn each box upside down and empty the contents to the floor. Categorise toys into new groups or into the groups that emerged when you were working on the shelves.

Finally, move on to any free-standing units and toy chests. Pull out the contents and identify the toy types. Check the surfaces of these units and around the back where toys tend to fall and get lost.

Here are a few of the categories that can be found in an organised toy room:

- Arts and crafts: paints, colours, crayons, colouring books, embellishments, coloured paper, glues, glitter, Play-Doh, finished art works

- Educational: sand, science kits, school items, supplies for children with special needs, wooden toys

- Large toys: blackboard, shopping trolley, kitchen, cash register, train set

- Costumes/dress-up

- Musical instruments

- Books

- DVDs

- Jigsaws and board games

- Computer games and electronics

- Soft toys, model animals, cars, etc.

- Lego

❷ DECLUTTER

We usually take the declutter stage as a separate step to allow you get into the flow of the work, take the pressure off making decisions from the word go and to allow your subconscious to think about things. However, if there are a lot of toys to contend with, it may be easier to throw out and donate as you categorise.

You may find that as you build categories you start to lose floor space, but by the time that happens you will start to see space opening up on the shelves or in the cabinets you started with. Space! Oh, joy and wonder!

In that case, find an empty shelf, cabinet, drawer or cubby hole and place a category of toys in it. This is a temporary home – a stop gap. It may well turn out that where you choose now is the perfect spot for this type of toy. However, that's not our focus at the moment. What we need to do now is simply categorise and declutter, but this gives us some breathing space to do so. We'll return to these spaces for a second sweep later.

It is essential when you are doing this that you keep one category to one shelf/ bin/drawer. You have already gone to the trouble of decluttering these toys, so don't give them a temporary home mixed in with other toys only to lose all the work you've done.

When you are deciding what to keep and what to let go, pull items right out and onto the floor. It's too difficult and time-consuming to declutter by looking into a box or toy chest or going along a shelf. Remove items fully. Sort them and declutter them sitting on the floor. From the floor you have a bird's eye view, allowing you to see clearly toys that might belong to each other, or bits of broken toys that you won't bother with at all. If you didn't have floor space to begin with, remember, use a nearby dining table or floor space to spread out on.

As you move to the toys on the floor, take it one wall at a time. As you go around the room, the messy side will start to reduce, the clean side will have items you want to keep and the bin or donation bags will be filling up by the minute!

Decluttering continues until you have worked the entire room.

The toy categories remaining will be either in a temporary home on a shelf or in a drawer, or they will be grouped on the floor. These are the toys you know you want to keep. There is no clutter any more, just toys with no home.

Now it's time to organise the toys into their final homes.

❸ ORGANISE

Once you have created categories and reduced the number of toys, it's time to assign each category to an available space in the room. When assigning homes to the toys, keep the organisation very simple. Always *decide on homes based on the kids' logic*, not on how you want it done.

Don't put toy chests in front of cabinets. Any storage that is low down is good for children's toys. If you place any obstacle in the way, even storage, all the storage behind it becomes unused and it's a waste of good storage. When placing items up on shelves or cabinets, always start with the priority items in your 'to keep' piles. Get those in place first. As soon as you start refilling any area, your space depletes. So home your priority items first. Keep the priority items down low, and closest to hand.

Lesser-used items or toy memorabilia go further out of reach, perhaps on higher shelves or at the back of cabinets.

If you lose space before all toys are up off your floor, you should only be left with the following:

- Very large toys that won't fit in storage anyway

- Toys you're unsure of

- Lower-priority toys.

The lower-priority toys and the toys you're unsure of (should you decide to keep them) will show you what storage you need.

LET SPACE BREATHE

You may have spare wall space and can buy another storage unit, but just because space opens up does not mean you have to use it and fill it. This also goes for cabinets and shelving. Having clear space allows the room to breathe. Let it sit. As you continue throughout the house, other uses for this clear space may emerge.

If you buy more storage, it's another thing to tidy and keep clean. Which is the lesser of two evils? Clear out these last few toys or buy the storage and maintain it? Remember, another storage product is not always the solution – decluttering is!

SHELVING/CUBBY HOLES

Categories that work well in cubby holes and on shelves are:

- SAND TRAY

- SCIENCE KITS

- SCHOOL ITEMS

- SUPPLIES FOR CHILDREN WITH SPECIAL NEEDS

- READING NOOK WITH BOOKS

- LARGE TOYS

- CASH REGISTER

- KITCHEN ITEMS/PLAY FOOD ITEMS

- ✓ BOOKS

- ✓ DVDS

- ✓ JIGSAWS

- ✓ GAMES

- ✓ COMPUTER GAMES AND ELECTRONICS

- ✓ TV/COMPUTER

SHALLOW DRAWERS

The following items work well in this space:

- ✓ ARTS AND CRAFTS
- ✓ PAINTS
- ✓ COLOURS
- ✓ CRAYONS
- ✓ COLOURING BOOKS
- ✓ EMBELLISHMENTS
- ✓ COLOURED PAPER
- ✓ GLUES, GLITTER

- ✓ ART CREATED
- ✓ SMALL TOY ZONE
- ✓ PLAY FOOD
- ✓ PLAY-DOH
- ✓ ANIMALS
- ✓ PEOPLE/FIGURINES
- ✓ CARS
- ✓ LEGO

FREE-STANDING DRAWER UNITS

If you own such a unit, look at the depth of the drawers and use them accordingly. For instance, shallow drawers are best for arts and crafts. Drawers of medium depth get slightly bigger toys or Lego. Deep drawers get computer games and electronics.

Remember, look at the size of the category, then match it with the size of the space available to you.

Try to keep one section of floor and wall space free. No posters on the walls, no toys on the floor. Just a little clear space will give you space in your head when you walk into the room. It will also be an area for the kids to play in and will give you an area to work in next time you need to do a toy room clear up (yes, I know that could be in two hours' time!).

Use the walls or alcoves for larger toys. Group the large toys together and line them up. This is their new home. Even though they're very big, keeping them together will make them look neater because they're corralled into one area. Large toys can take up a lot of space, so be ruthless with what you're keeping.

CORNERS OF THE ROOM

Be creative with the corners of a toy room. If your children love reading, create a reading zone and place their little chairs, a bookshelf or a small desk here. If they love theatre, create a small performance zone. Place a rail on the diagonal between two walls and hang curtains on it to create a small stage. Or simply gather their musical instruments into this corner. Add their costumes and dressing-up accessories into the corner too so they have everything in one corner to play pretend.

❹ STORAGE

When storing toys, match the size of the item with the size of available space. For example, jigsaws and books may fit in a container, but are you getting the maximum use out of the container space? Assign toys to storage that invites using the product to its fullest, not just because the toy happens to fit.

Choose the size of containers carefully. Small items such as figurines, Lego and dolls' clothes need a small container, which may seem logical. But what often happens is that several of the same-sized containers are bought for all toys. If the container is too big for a particular type of toy, other items get thrown in on top of them and everything gets mixed up and lost. Which is why it's so important to know what you have, what you're keeping and the size of it before any storage is bought.

ALWAYS DECIDE ON HOMES BASED ON THE KIDS' LOGIC, NOT ON HOW YOU WANT IT DONE.

NO STORAGE NEEDED

Games, jigsaws and books can usually hold their own and don't necessarily need storage.

SHALLOW CONTAINERS WITHOUT LIDS

Small containers are used for small toys. Containers are ideal for toys with bits that can become dispersed (Lego, bricks, tea sets, etc.). I would avoid buying boxes or containers with lids for toy room storage. While it may look great for you, children will, inevitably, not replace the lids. They'll pull the lid off to get at the toys and the lid will be lost for ever. For tidying up, we want to make it as easy as possible for the kids to put things away.

No lids makes cleaning the toy room easier for you, too. With open containers, well labelled, you can simply pick up and pop toys back where they belong. Always remember ease of access for the kids – more so for clean-up time than play time!

MEDIUM-DEPTH CONTAINERS WITHOUT LIDS

Containers are also essential for all computer games, accessories and electronics such as cables, wires, consoles, remote controls, etc.

DEEP CONTAINERS WITHOUT LIDS

Doctors and nurses sets, trains and train track are all bulky and so need deeper containers or baskets.

STORAGE BENCHES

Benches with storage inside can be a great addition to a toy room. This gives a lovely seating area but also space to home toys.

TOY BINS ON WHEELS

These can be rolled out into the middle of the room, toys picked out and played with and then when they're done the storage is right next to them to encourage them to put the toys away. All that's left is to roll the storage back into place.

COLOURFUL TUBS

Large colourful tubs are good for teddy bears and musical instruments.

MINI WARDROBES

If your children love to dress up, is there space for a mini wardrobe, or even a little rail? If not, a toy chest can hold costumes and all the little accessories that come with them.

As mentioned above, we assign a section of floor space to large toys such as a blackboard, shopping trolley, kitchen cooker, buggy or pram. To make this space work even better, use bright tape and mark out a 'parking space' for each toy. Take a photo of the toy and stick the photo on the ground to indicate the assigned parking space. The kids will love putting their toys away into the parking space!

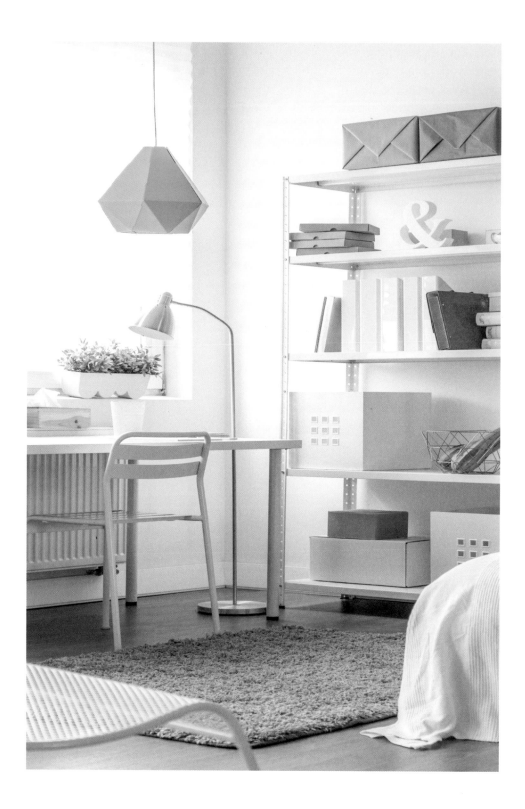

15

SPARE ROOMS

•

I LOVE CLEARING SPARE ROOMS. YOU CAN GET A
GOOD RESULT REALLY QUICKLY IN THESE ROOMS.
HONESTLY, YOU CAN! *THIS ROOM IS NOT AS
IMPOSSIBLE AS YOU THINK.*

•

During a home assessment, I'm usually brought
into this room last. It's the room that causes most
embarrassment, the 'worst' room; clients hate it
and are mortified to show it to anyone.

•

Like decluttering it, they're procrastinating — putting off bringing me to it. I copped on to this tactic pretty quickly, so now I always visit this room first.

THE PROBLEM

- Items not put back in the attic.
- Items not put away following a move.
- Attic is full and there's nowhere else to store the items.
- You don't have an attic and this is a substitute attic.
- The room was mid-renovation when you got side-tracked.
- You're unsure what the room's function will be.
- The room is full, you're unsure what's in there and no room or time to clear it.

THE AIM

First of all, we have to figure out once and for all what you are going to use the room for. Think of the possibilities. No really, *think*. What do you want to use it for? What do you *need* to use it for? It's always better and more motivating if you declutter a room with a purpose. You need to know what you're working towards.

Is the goal for this room an office? A guest room? A craft/hobby room? A place to relax? A teenager's den? A walk-in wardrobe? A substitute attic?

Decide what function or functions this room is going to have before you begin.

BEFORE YOU BEGIN

If you are having issues with the rest of your house, may I present to you your real problem? Spare room, meet client; client, meet spare room. This room is the juggernaut in your home. It's not the only one but it's a big obstacle to getting the rest of the house sorted.

Why? It's usually got excellent storage in the forms of wardrobes, shelves and drawers that are not being used well. Most items here should have gone out or up to the attic months ago. So you're procrastinating, and this will be a reflection of how other things are dealt with in the rest of the rooms in the home.

'But it's full,' I hear you say. Well, I'm often asked to work on a client's kitchen, or bedroom or utility room, and during the assessment they'll show me the spare room but it's not the priority. The other rooms are priorities because they see that mess every day and they want the rooms they're actually living in to work well for them. However, I'll invariably suggest working here. Maybe not first, but to see real change in the home, it has to be done sometime. As I said, it's your juggernaut.

But don't panic; it's always easier than you think. There are several reasons for that. First, items in here are so old that you won't believe you've kept these things for so long, so it's easy to let them go. Or, second, there's not as much stuff as you thought: the room itself is small and there's usually furniture that is actually taking up most of the space. Third, the storage in this room is never used to its maximum. Therefore, even if you do need to keep items, if you have cleared and reorganised the space that a wardrobe or chest of drawers gives you, lo and behold, these items will find a home. Better yet, it's often a combination of all three. And with some elbow grease and better organisation, the room will be clear.

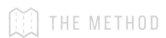 ## THE METHOD

So let's get going! When tackling this room, start with the floor, then the bed, followed by wardrobes and shelving.

❶ CATEGORISE

The categories often found in a spare room are:

- Books
- CDs, DVDs, computer games
- Arts and crafts
- Towels and bed linen
- Excess cushions, throws
- Sleeping bags, mattresses
- Travel/holiday gear
- Christmas/Easter decorations
- Old baby and kids' clothes
- Wedding presents
- Old school books
- Old kids' art
- Old toiletries
- Memorabilia – yours, your partner's, your kids', your parents'

- Clothes, shoes, handbags, coats
- Large items – cots, luggage, Christmas tree, old lamps, ornaments, tents
- Photographs, photo frames, art
- Random cardboard boxes full of items of unknown origin
- Headboards
- Items to be sold
- Items from the in-laws
- Items from deceased parents or in-laws
- Items to be returned to others
- Hoover/iron/ironing board
- Electronics, wires, cables

And money – lots and lots of spare coins (told you you'd save money!) with a random lost wedding ring thrown in to keep you on your toes! I reckon that's enough for one room, don't you?

THE FLOOR

Begin to categorise what you find. If you have an attic, ignore everything else and just search for attic items; items you should have put up there ages ago but didn't get around to. These are easy to identify and it gets you started on this process. Continue to group items. Group luggage together, toys together, spare mattresses, pillows and duvets together.

THE BED

Examine the items on it. Place like with like. Remember, imagine the bed as a grid of squares, each square for a category of items. Keep the items in their categories on a certain section of the bed.

THE WARDROBE

The wardrobe(s) in a spare room are the secret to your success. You have to get these working well. Each rail, each cubby hole and each shelf will get a job to do, even if that job is yet to be determined.

If you have more than one wardrobe in this room and clothes in both, bring all clothes into one of them. Create a zone for clothes. The other wardrobe is now free to act as storage space.

Taking one cubby hole at a time, empty the contents. You will more than likely find items that slot into categories you have on the bed. If so, add to those categories and create new categories if you need to. If there's no room on the bed, use the floor. Place the items neatly where other clutter will not be accidentally added to them. This is only temporary, so don't worry.

If you run out of space on the floor or bed, take one category and assign it to a shelf, as we did with toys. This is merely to create space. Do not mistake this for creating a home for it. It may well turn out to be the perfect spot, but right now the focus is on decluttering and creating space.

THE CHEST OF DRAWERS

Take it one drawer at a time. Literally toss everything onto the floor and sort it. Take each item at a time and decide on its fate. Is it for the bin, recycling, donation? Does it belong to an existing category, or is it an item that will create a new category?

SHELVING

Shelves in a spare room are very often not completely full. Some shelves are full of toys or books, but then there are other shelves that only have a scattering of loose sunglasses, hair clips, the odd picture frame, old cassette tapes all dotted around them.

Simply tidy the books and toys – they're too big to remove, but do corral them together. There is no point removing books from shelves to add them to your book category on the floor or bed. The books are going to stay on the shelves. So look at the bed or floor, and if there are books there, add them to the shelves now that there is space.

Then focus on the random clutter. Can you add any items to the categories already created?

❷ DECLUTTER

Taking a category at a time, decide what goes and what stays. Because many items end up in this room as a result of an overflow from another room, tips to declutter items such as clothes, toys, stationery or arts and crafts can be found in the other chapters.

Here's some other decluttering to consider.

LARGE FURNITURE

Large furniture in a spare room can create a barrier to organising it. Now is the time to really look at the pieces of furniture and decide if you need them. They may be taking up a huge amount of space.

For instance, if you have two lockers, one on either side of the bed, can you get rid of one? Or both? Do you really need the bed itself?

Most people like to keep a bed in the spare room for visitors. However, very often when I probe a little bit, I find that in fact it's rare that visitors need to stay over; and if they do have to, there are other alternatives in the home to accommodate them. Ask yourself if you really need the bed. Would it be beneficial to remove it altogether?

If so, then start making plans and taking action now to move it out. If you're going to sell it, get it online. Use your time wisely. Have the sale of the bed or other furniture working away in the background as you continue decluttering. Hopefully, by the time the room is decluttered, the furniture will be sold and you'll have the space to finish the organisation and design of the room.

DIFFICULT ITEMS

Some of the most difficult items are those from deceased relatives or items that you've inherited. Decluttering someone else's possessions isn't easy. It's even harder if your own stuff is muddled with theirs. Make it easier on yourself and clearly divide up what is yours and what was theirs. What you can do now, and what will take longer.

There are two projects in one here, so try to separate them out. Can you section part of the room and create a hub for these more difficult items? Then one half of the room contains inherited items to be assessed; the other half is where the new spare room will emerge.

Clear the room of everything that *isn't* considered part of the 'inherited' zone. Once that is done, the only disorganisation to tackle is the inherited items. This will be easier now the rest of the room works better. You will now know that everything you are looking at is exactly what you should be looking at. You don't have clothes or toys or old school work in on top of past papers, old ornaments, historical documents, etc.

You also have space to pull these items out and look through them. You'll have space to walk into the room and manoeuvre. This will not only help you practically but it will give you head space to deal with the more emotionally charged items.

ITEMS FOR THE ATTIC

Declutter items for the attic last. This bit will probably be straightforward; everything in this category will be going straight up to the attic. Therefore, go through the other categories that are more difficult to make decisions on first. Once that's done, return to this easier category.

❸ ORGANISE

While you may have grand plans to convert the spare room or return it to its former glory as a guest room or office, that can be hard to do completely. A lot of items in this room take longer to move out because you may want to sell them or give them to a family member. It may be another few months before that happens.

With that in mind, if you have to put items back in, remember your zones. Use one corner for all your items you plan to sell. Use another corner for all the items to be given to someone you know.

After that, use the storage available to the maximum – under the bed, upper wardrobes, deep drawers, bookshelves.

As we discussed earlier in this chapter, removing large furniture may help you, depending on your goal for this room. If you choose to keep the bed, make it work to your advantage. Can you add drawers or under-bed storage? If it already has drawers, each drawer will get a specific storage job to do. Categories that are good for under the bed include:

- LUGGAGE

- SEASONAL CLOTHES

- TOWELS

- BED LINEN

- MEMORABILIA

- WEDDING GIFTS

- OLD BABY AND KIDS' CLOTHES

THE WARDROBE

Use the upper shelves for less used items. Categories that work well in these spaces include:

- SEASONAL CLOTHES

- SEASONAL DECORATIONS

- LUGGAGE

- MEMORABILIA

- BAGS AND RUCKSACKS

If the upper shelves are too narrow for large bulky items, use the bottom of the wardrobe. However, as said before, make sure that long flowing clothes are not draping over the items here. This will look messy and won't make it easy to get items in and out of that space – which will eventually lead back to clutter.

Cubby holes need to be well thought out. Big bulky items are best stored here because it is a big, bulky space. Items that work well here include:

- ✓ CHUNKY SWEATERS

- ✓ BOOKS, DVDS

- ✓ BOARD GAMES

- ✓ BULKY OFFICE SUPPLIES, E.G. PRINTER PAPER, LEVER ARCH FOLDERS

- ✓ MEMORABILIA

If you are using the cubby holes for smaller items, place containers of a similar size to the cubby hole inside them to contain everything. For example, a large plastic container the size of a standard wardrobe cubby hole could hold a lot of loose Lego.

But be warned: if there's a lot of empty space in the container, you run the risk of people throwing anything inside it merely because there's space. So ensure that the container is clearly labelled and it's very obvious what the container's job is. If you don't, lo and behold, instead of just a cubby hole with random clutter in it, you'll have a storage box inside a cubby hole with random clutter in it.

If you have a wardrobe with a double rail (a high one and a midway one), the lower rail is often not needed. If you can arrange your clothes on the upper rail, remove the lower one, store it at the back and use all this lower space for storage.

CHEST OF DRAWERS

If the bottom of any of the drawers is broken, consider the drawer null and void. While you could repair it, I suspect that, because it's in the spare room, DIY on such an item is more time-consuming than it's worth. In that instance, I would be considering whether to keep the unit at all.

If you are down a drawer, it's even more important to plan the chest's use well. Items that work well here include:

- ✓ CLOTHING

- ✓ BABY CLOTHES

- ✓ BABY PARAPHERNALIA – TOILETRIES, TOWELLING, LINEN

- ✓ ARTS AND CRAFTS

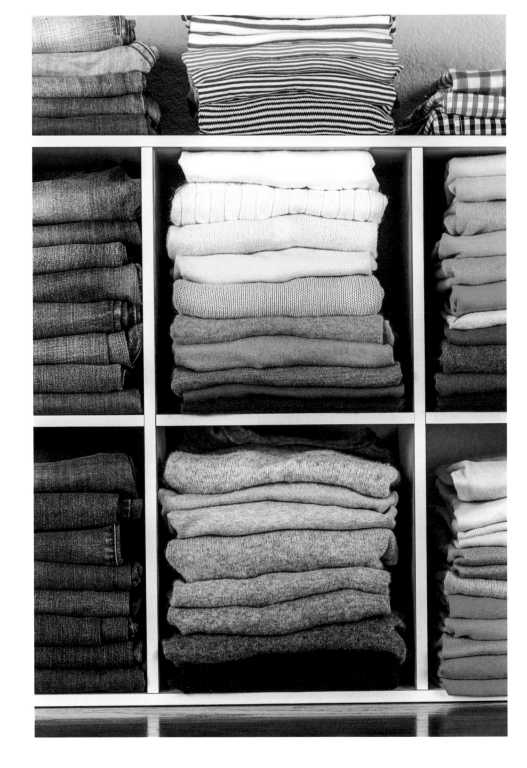

✓ **BED LINEN**

✓ **TOWELS**

✓ **STATIONERY**

SHELVING

Begin by placing items that are normally found on a shelf here, such as books, DVDs, CDs, games and jigsaws. You may already have started that during the declutter stage. Place items of top priority first, on shelves at eye level. Lesser-used items go on top and bottom shelves. Items for children are also designated to the bottom shelves.

Items that are strong and heavy enough to keep them steady are unlikely to topple over and become untidy. Those items are good for shelves – chunky knitted jumpers, magazines in magazine files, towels, bed linen, for example.

If you only have smaller items to home, use matching containers along the length of the shelves and place the small items inside.

If you have any photos in frames or ornaments to home, use the shelves for these items but space them neatly. Remember, you don't have to fill every inch of shelving just because you have space.

❹ STORAGE

What storage you use in this room will depend on whether you are going to keep it as a room for additional storage, use it as a guest room or completely redesign it as an office. See Chapter 13 for ideas on storage for an additional bedroom and Chapter 16 for ideas about storage for an office.

If you wish to keep it as storage, in lieu of an attic or as an extension to one, here are some suggestions about storage that will help keep it organised.

TACKLE BOXES

Tackle boxes are fantastic for a whole host of small items from stationery to toys, decorations to batteries and light bulbs.

STORAGE FOR SEASONAL DECORATIONS

Containers that are divided inside are perfect for Christmas tree ornaments. You can find solutions for storing Christmas wreaths and lights online. For a simple storage solution for lights, place each set into their own bag – a large clear sandwich or grocery bag. Then put all the bags of lights into a box. Using an empty roll of kitchen paper per set also works. Or you could try the empty spool from electrical wire.

Fabric storage bags work well for Christmas decorations because they can often fall out of shape over the years and won't fit well in their original boxes. Fabric gives more flexibility.

STORAGE FOR GIFT WRAP AND CARDS

Standard storage boxes work perfectly fine. Use one box solely for cards and another box for tags, ribbons, bags and folded wrapping paper.

If you have recently bought a new pillow that came in a plastic bag, recycle this bag for large rolls of wrapping paper. They fit perfectly.

You can also find containers specifically made for gift wrap organisation online, and they can look amazing.

SPECIALISED STORAGE

Wedding dresses need to be protected in a pH neutral container. Use acid-free tissue paper to wrap the dress.

Out-of-season clothing or memorabilia such as baby clothes will also benefit from being stored in acid-free tissue. Use cedar blocks or cedar-lined storage to deter insects. Plastic storage is okay, but make sure it is clean and there is no trapped moisture. Storage boxes made of acid-free paper are good, as are clean suitcases.

Make sure all garments are washed and clean before storage to kill any insects that may be in them. All garments need clean, cool, dry and dark conditions.

Consider storage with handles if you are pulling heavy boxes or boxes from a height. And consider storage on wheels, if you need to push heavy boxes underneath something.

DRAWER DIVIDERS

Use drawer dividers in drawers to corral small items for hobbies and crafting. These items are tidier and more useful in small containers or drawer dividers:

- ✓ **PENCILS AND PAINTS**

- ✓ **MATERIALS – VARIOUS SIZES**

- ✓ **THREADS/EMBROIDERY**

- ✓ **FELT**

- ✓ **SEWING**

- ✓ **FABRIC MARKERS AND DYES**

OFFICE STORAGE

Storage for offices is described in the next chapter.

GUEST ROOM STORAGE

Storage for bedrooms is described in Chapter 13.

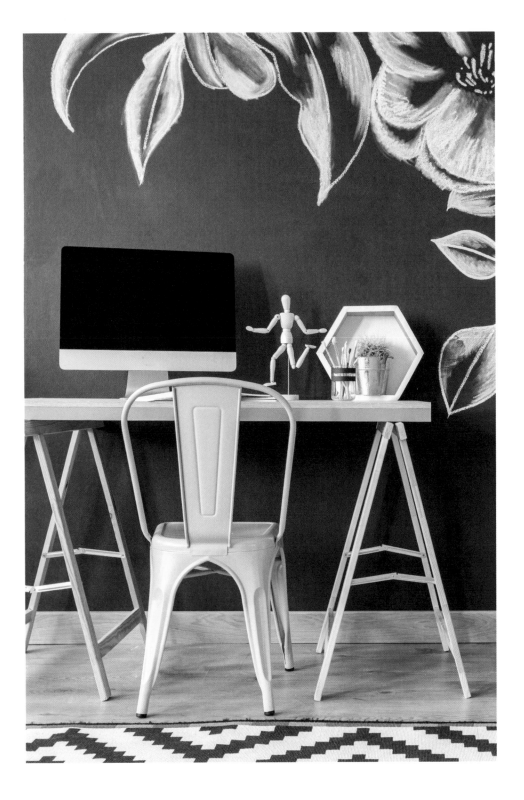

16

HOME OFFICES

·

WHETHER YOU ARE WORKING FROM A HOME OFFICE, CORNER OFFICE OR A CUBICLE, GETTING THE SPACE ORGANISED WILL INJECT ENERGY AND INSPIRATION.

·

Clearing clutter from the area that is to bring you success – financially, professionally and personally – is a no-brainer for me. As you clear it, new opportunities have space to enter.

·

Taking time out to organise office space can be difficult. You can't work effectively here, which drains your time management, yet you need time out in order to fix the organisation. It's a vicious circle.

Offices need to function well. If they're organised properly they can be a source of great inspiration. At home, an office space can be a fantastic addition that can really ease your stress and help your work/life balance.

THE PROBLEM

- The original office has outgrown its space

- No room to work

- Variety of items, from paperclips to magazines, all without homes

- Piles of un-filed and disorganised paperwork

- Unopened letters

- Tangled cables and wires, covered in dust, losing their protective cover and no longer safe

- No floor space

- Not enough storage

- Sharing space with other people

- Sharing the space with other functions of the house

- The space is depressing and needs refurbishment

THE AIM

This room can serve a number of purposes, or even be a multifunctional space. Some examples are a dedicated work space for your career, for your business, to study or to run a busy family.

- To create a space that is functional yet comfortable and inspiring.

- To organise it so that it can be decorated.

- To organise it so that you can start a business.

- To organise it so that a new employee can be hired.

- To create a calm study area for a teenager or for your own part-time study.

- To facilitate a hobby.

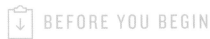

BEFORE YOU BEGIN

If you have a home office, keeping it organised helps keep work and home life separate and balanced. Even if you don't have a home office, creating an office zone helps you control your work items, your time and productivity.

Nowadays many homes set up a home office without thinking if they actually need one or not.

For instance, you may decide to have one to accommodate the kids' studying. However, kids often prefer to work at the kitchen table, where they are near the rest of the family. Others – teenagers especially – work better in their bedrooms. You may have set up a home office because you used to work from home, but perhaps you no longer do so. You may have hobbies, such as crafting, for which you thought a home office would be useful.

During the nineties, a dedicated room for a home office was the norm. Nowadays, as we move more online, a simple desk, chair and lamp can suffice for an office. Some people consider a laptop and phone an adequate office.

All of which is why taking time out to consider the need for a home office is important for the workings of this room and the overall organisation of your home.

ORGANISING AN OFFICE IN AN EXISTING ROOM

Often, the home office is part of another room, maybe in the corner of the living room or the toy room or your bedroom. It can be difficult to keep the office tidy and functioning if it is sharing a room. Clear boundaries are required when splitting a room up to accommodate an office. Try the following solutions.

- Create a closet office. Build the office into a cabinet that can be closed at the end of the day. There are hundreds of ideas on this on Pinterest and they can be functional and very beautiful.

- Use the back of a couch, a bookcase or other large piece of furniture to create a divide to separate work and home.

- If you cannot create a divide, keep office and home items separate by zoning the storage furniture. For example, in a guest room, use the chest of drawers for all items pertaining to the guest, the bedroom and other home storage, and use the wardrobe for your office. Remove the rail, add in shelving and keep all your office and business supplies there. If you need the wardrobe for other things, perhaps you could fit a large cabinet in the room that would accommodate your office items.

Either way, *do not mix work and pleasure*. Use the storage and furniture you have to distinguish the two functions in the room.

PAPERWORK

In this chapter we deal with organising everything in the office except paperwork. Paper is the most difficult thing to organise and keep organised, so I've dedicated the next chapter to it.

I'm talking about documents, paper you use to create your to-dos and paper to file. When you find that sort of paper, simply place the paperwork together in one pile.

When paper is mentioned in this chapter it means actual paper – coloured card, printer paper, letterheads, etc. – not documents or files.

PERSONAL ITEMS

If your office is particularly messy, I suggest removing all non-office paraphernalia until the office is organised – candles, ornaments, frames, trinkets belonging to you, your kids or parents – it should all be removed so that you are only left with office items to focus on.

Later, when the office is organised, you might consider new decor and it is at that stage when we can reintroduce more personal items to add some personality.

OFFICES
ORGANISED
PROPERLY CAN
BE A SOURCE
OF GREAT
INSPIRATION.

The best way to get to grips with an office is to block out a chunk of time, as you would a holiday, and blitz the area in one go. Drip-feeding organisation into this space just won't cut it. It is the one space where you need to rip the bandage off quickly and get it over with.

❶ CATEGORISE

In the office, I split the work between organising the desk and organising the rest of the room.

THE DESK

You have a desk space you need to work at, but it is covered in paper and you don't know what belongs to what. There is a range of stationery, media and technology that you're sure is now damaged and some torn-out pages from magazines. There are gift vouchers, business cards, loyalty cards for coffee, and receipts. It's a mess. You hate working there. Every time you clear it, it soon gets messy again.

Now, you may ask why I'm insisting you start with the desk when the rest of the room is a mess. This is because I know your time is precious. You may be decluttering your office while your kids are in crèche or in between Skype calls. Or you may have taken holiday time to get this done. So, while I want you to get started on the room, I also want you to be able to get back to work here as soon as possible and then declutter the rest of the room.

Also, the practice of decluttering and tidying the desk will fall into your maintenance routine later on. In the future, if you're ever stuck for time, clearing the desk will make you feel better and give you the sense that the room is more organised. It is also a lesson in 'good enough'. You don't need this room to be perfect in order to work here. It is possible to have a clear working space on one side and your decluttering to-dos on the other.

So let's get started.

STEP I. PAPER

Gather up all the loose bits of paper on your desk. Even if you need to filter through those bits of paper later on, even if they don't belong to each other, pile them together. When you get the desk clear, if you have no other work to go through, you can take this pile of paper and whittle through it. For now, leave the papers in a neat pile to one side of your desk.

STEP 2. **TECHNOLOGY**

Now look at technology. Wrap up wires and cables, gather together disks, CDs, equipment, USB sticks, etc. Bundle those together to one side of the desk.

STEP 3. **STATIONERY**

Next, gather up pens, staplers, scissors, paperclips, etc. If you have drawers or containers for these things, use them. Put the stationery away. Even if the drawer you are putting the items into is a mess it doesn't matter. Put the items away. Like the pile of paper, if you have time, you can declutter the stationery drawer later. For now, we need a desk to work from.

This is tidying without worrying about decluttering or organisation. You are not going to get it completely clear. Additional to-dos will emerge. However, you will clear a working space for yourself.

Place your computer or laptop in the middle of the desk. To one side, depending on whether you are right- or left-handed, have a clear space to take notes. Have some stationery within arm's reach. Hook up the printer.

Now, if you get nothing else done in the room, you can work from your desk.

This practice here will carry forward into the future. When you have the room fully organised, your desk will inevitably become messy because it is a working desk. When you use it, no matter how organised the room around you is, it will become a mess again. Now you have a way of organising it quickly so you can get back to your daily hustle.

THE REST OF THE ROOM

The desk usually reflects the typical categories found in an office. The categories that have emerged, such as paper, technology and stationery, will remain the primary categories as you move through the room.

Your next job is to examine the drawers in the desk and the shelves above it, if any. Add items to the categories created or form new ones.

Next move to the floor. You will need this clear so there is room to manoeuvre.

Use an area of the floor to spread your categories. If you have a bed or a couch in the room, you might like to use this instead. Remember, we imagine a grid and place different categories in each box of the grid.

From the floor, move to the furniture in the room – shelves, drawer units, cabinets. Empty them out and continue to build your categories.

FILING CABINETS

If you do have a paper problem, the chances are it's because:

- Storage is full and so there's nowhere for paper to go.

- You have trouble getting rid of paper.

- Both of the above.

Tips are given in the next chapter for getting rid of paper and how to organise paper inside a filing cabinet.

However, sometimes filing cabinets contain stationery and technology too, or some drawers are only half full. The filing cabinet is not being used to its maximum. For now, as we are looking at all non-paper items, remove anything that's not paper from the cabinets and examine the contents. Categorise items, adding them to categories already created or creating new ones.

For example, you may find supplies for your camera, which you have not found so far, so start a new 'camera' category. Or you may find a ream of printer paper. You can add this to the broad 'stationery' category or you might like to start a separate 'paper' category, to which you will later add laminated paper and photo paper.

As we are forever writing notes to ourselves or starting a new notebook every time we want to get organised there are usually random scraps of paper, Post-it notes and half-empty notebooks scattered round an office.

If you find Post-its with notes on them as you go, staple them to an A4 piece of paper. Group all your notebooks together. Staple scraps of paper together too. Keep all the notes you've written to yourself in their own category.

With that, here are some more categories that are found in an office:

- DOCUMENTS OF VARYING DEGREES OF IMPORTANCE: to-do notes, notes on Post-its, notes on random pieces of paper, short-term filing, long-term filing, items to archive

- MULTIMEDIA: iPads, voice recorders, presentation equipment, phones

- WIRES AND CABLES for current (and past) equipment

- LARGE EQUIPMENT: computers, laptops, screens, printers, hard drives, laminators

- CAMERAS: camera cards, wires, lenses

- WRITING MATERIALS: pens, pencils, colours, highlighters

- NOTEBOOKS

- SMALL STATIONERY ITEMS: paperclips, bulldog clips, stapler, hole punch

- LARGE STATIONERY ITEMS: plastic pockets, folders

- PAPER: envelopes (various sizes), printer paper, coloured card, laminator paper

- BUSINESS STATIONERY: paper, envelopes, compliment slips, business cards

- READING MATERIAL: magazines, newspapers, supplier brochures, marketing brochures, research papers

- TRADE SHOW PARAPHERNALIA

- BOOKS

Corralling these items into broad categories is the first step to taking control of your environment.

You can follow the categories above, or you might consider categories that follow themes, for example:

- Items I need for the next TRADE SHOW

- Items I need for the next WORKSHOP

- Items I need for the next CHARITY EVENT

- Items I need when I'M WORKING FROM HOME

- Items I need when I'M WORKING WITH A CLIENT

Or a mixture of both. For example, the category 'Items I need for the next trade show' might include a selection of writing instruments, business stationery, marketing brochures, etc., but you would also have a stock of all these items elsewhere too.

Sorting the office is going to take a few sessions. At each session tackle a different piece of furniture.

HERE ARE SOME FINAL TIPS

- Along the way, you will find receipts. Have an A4 envelope to hand, and put receipts in there as you go. You will sort them when you tackle paperwork.

- You will also find money, from coins to foreign currency. Put this in a container, clear bag or wallet.

- If you find random phone numbers as you go, detail them all on one piece of paper and return to them later.

- You will find passwords too. Keep them all on one piece of paper. This isn't the most secure place, but they weren't too safe on a Post-it stuck to the back of a 1981 copy of *Time* magazine either. Or maybe they were. Either way, keep passwords together and we'll find a system later.

- Keep a piece of paper to one side to test whether pens work as you go along. If they don't, out they go.

❷ DECLUTTER

Now we have created categories for the items in the room, it's time to make some space. Taking each category, reduce what you own.

NO-BRAINERS

Get rid of the following:

- ✓ **DUPLICATES AND PHOTOCOPIES.** If you really need a second copy, you can get it again. If the duplicate was for someone else, add it to the 'belongs elsewhere' pile.

- ✓ **OUT-OF-DATE BROCHURES.**

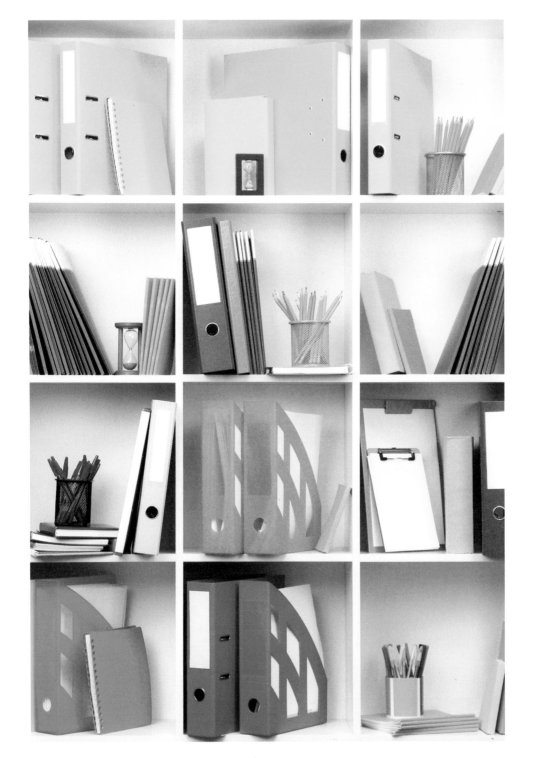

✓ **OLD MAGAZINES AND NEWSPAPERS**. They may have been kept for research purposes, but if they're 8, 10, 15 years old now, I think research may have moved on.

✓ **ANYTHING BROKEN** – pens, staplers, bent paperclips, suspension files.

NOTEBOOKS AND LOOSE NOTES

Now start to flick through loose notes and throw out as much as you can. This may take a little while, so give yourself time. A lot of notes were probably written quite a while ago. If you can't decipher the writing, get rid of it. If you haven't needed it by now, you probably don't need it. If it's important, it will come back again – either via the person or situation, or your brain will jog your memory.

Flick through notebooks. If they are only half full, you can rip out the pages you have written on and keep the notebook.

Any notes you are keeping form to-dos. They are either tasks you wanted or needed to do, or they contain information you need to log and file somewhere. They will be dealt with when you organise your paperwork.

WIRES AND CABLES

It can cause anxiety to throw out wires and cables when you're not 100 per cent sure what they belong to. So keep out the wires for the printer, cameras, laminators, Apple products, laptops and phones that you currently use. Keep the rest in a separate box to declutter in more detail at a later stage. There is no point wasting time wondering about these wires now. Knowing they are not current or used for the main pieces of equipment is knowledge enough for now. You have bigger fish to fry.

STATIONERY

If you can quickly check whether a pen works, do so. Don't waste valuable organising time spending 15 minutes checking a box of pens and markers. There are many, many boxes of pens and markers out there. If they are very old – as they tend to be – there's a good chance they won't be working and should be thrown out.

When you categorise the stationery together, you may like to split the category further, giving each family member some stationery. This works if you have a lot and the kids are of school-going age. If these situations don't apply to you, let go of old, broken, multiple pieces of stationery. There are few things more frustrating than a pair of scissors or stapler that doesn't work.

LARGE FURNITURE AND EQUIPMENT

Old laptops, broken printers, discontinued versions all need to go. It's now or never. Arrange for the laptops to be wiped, if you wish, as part of your decluttering stage. If you wish to sell anything, create a 'for sale' pile and dedicate an evening to photographing and uploading everything online. Instead of leaving this until the end, items can be selling as you continue to organise the room. They take up too much space, so move them out.

❸ ORGANISE

At this stage you have reduced what you own, and the things you are keeping are in category bundles. Now let's look at the space you have in the office and where you will re-home each category.

THE DESK

Your desk surface helps you work. It is not a storage solution. There may be storage within it, but the surface is for work. This area is for your computer, mouse and some space to spread out. So try to have as little as possible on the desk so that you can use it to work on rather than as a surface to store office supplies.

Having this clear space allows you to spread out for any reading, writing or research you may be doing. It's also important ergonomically. You should be able to place your elbow on the desk and stretch your lower arm out straight to the keyboard. This reduces the chance of repetitive strain injury.

If you have to use the desktop as storage – for stationery, magazine files, in/out trays – keep these items to one side or in the corners so that you have as much desk space available as possible. Think of a semi-circle when you place items on the desk. Items closest to you are those you need most often. Items you use less often are placed further away. Think out and up. Use the outer extremities of the desk, shelves above, cabinets to the right and left rather than the desk surface itself.

Finally, feng shui experts recommend that your office chair is not placed so that your back is to the door. Try not to face the wall either.

I regularly see drawer units on wheels, and they are often full. Those units are great for wires, stationery, school supplies, arts and crafts. They aren't good for any level of paperwork or for filing it. If you have these units, use them for small items only.

Bookshelves and cabinets are a good bet. You will get a lot on them and they will take a range of different-shaped items. If you can, choose shelves or cabinets that are the full height of the wall to maximise the available vertical space. Assign a different category to each shelf. For example, you could plan a six-shelf cabinet like this:

- Shelf 1 (bottom shelf): laptop cases, briefcases

- Shelf 2: spare stationery

- Shelf 3: current stationery

- Shelf 4: marketing material

- Shelf 5: books, DVDs, CDs

- Shelf 6 (top shelf): photos, photo albums, photo boxes.

Once you lay out the categories on the shelving, you can then add storage to streamline the organisation.

Filing cabinets don't have to exclusively hold your important documents. Suspension files are good storage for some stationery that will store horizontally, for example A4 envelopes, A4 labels, spare paper folders, plastic pockets, folder dividers, coloured card, laminator paper, photo paper, printer paper.

These were initially created for catching post as it came in. Now they can be used in many different ways. Some of them come stacked in three. If you choose that, as always, give each tray a job. For example:

	SUGGESTION 1	SUGGESTION 2	SUGGESTION 3	SUGGESTION 4
TOP	Paper in	To-dos	Printer paper	Notebooks
MIDDLE	Paper in progress	To file	Photo paper	Magazines
BOTTOM	Paper out	To throw out	Coloured paper	Cut-outs for inspiration

LET THERE BE LIGHT

We all know that poor lighting causes eye strain and headaches and can have a negative effect on productivity. The best light is natural light, so bear this in mind when you are deciding where to place or move your desk.

Then consider your artificial lighting. A desk light that shines directly on your work can be a huge help on dark winter days.

The colour white can also help the light in your office as it will reflect any available light for you. It also gives the impression that there is more space, which can be hugely beneficial in how we feel about the space we are working in.

WIRES AND CABLES

When you start to see some organisation appear in the room, the wires and cables you have plugged in will stick out like a sore thumb. Through tiredness or sheer lack of enthusiasm you might find it quicker to fix the wires without unplugging the equipment. You will move one wire, which will intertwine with another and then you'll end up having to fix that. You might not want to, but it is much quicker (and safer) to unplug everything, untangle it and plug it all in again. It'll also look much better.

PASSWORDS

I'm no IT expert, but here are some tips on how best to protect passwords.

✓ **DON'T USE THE SAME PASSWORD FOR EVERYTHING.**

✓ **CHANGE THEM PERIODICALLY.**

✓ **KEEP ONE MASTER PASSWORD AND STORE THE REST.**

✓ **PROTECT YOUR COMPUTER WITH ANTI-VIRUS SOFTWARE.**

✓ **KEEP SOFTWARE UP TO DATE.**

Photos are so important to us, yet nowadays they live in our phones or on our laptops for years. There will be generations of children who have no albums to flick through and reminisce. Organising photos is a project all by itself, and one you could have in the back of your mind to tackle down the road. Don't even think that while you're organising an office or paperwork that you have time for photographs as well. You don't. Organise rooms first, then when you're living in organisational bliss, you can sort photos at your leisure.

As you tackle the office, you will find photos between sheets of paper, on surfaces and in cupboards. So you need a solution in place to hold the photos until you get to your photography project. A quick and super-easy solution is to get a box. As you find photos, in they go. Put a nice label on the front. It's very easy to become distracted and start looking at the photos and reliving memories. Don't succumb to this. Keep organising. You can enjoy looking through the photos when the office is finished later.

Once you have tackled your office and paper, all the photos you found along the way will be stored neatly in a box, ready for you to take on your photo project and start creating albums and keeping memories alive!

Categorise — *Sort the photos one by one. Categories and sub-categories will emerge, e.g. 'Holidays – France', 'Events – Jane's Debs', 'Family – Ben's 21st'. Write each sub-category on a Post-it and place it on top of the bundle of photos. Hold them together with an elastic band. Place the photos in an envelope with the overall category written on it. This will keep them organised and together until you get proper storage for them.*

The digital categorisation of photos should reflect the categorisation created for physical photos. For example, you have some physical photos and some digital photos of Jane's debs. The bundle of photos is categorised with other family events, such as weddings and christenings. Therefore, on your computer you would also have a folder called 'Events', in which there would be sub-folders entitled 'Jane's debs', 'Tom's christening', etc.

Creating categories with your physical photos will make it easier to manage your digital ones as you will simply reflect on your computer what you created and organised in real life.

Declutter *Don't keep any poor-quality, blurred or unwanted photos. They will only cause clutter in your home and/or on your computer.*

Purchasing an external hard drive is essential not only for protecting your photos but also for keeping your computer files organised. Once the folders of photos are moved to the external hard drive they can be deleted off your computer, freeing up space.

Organise *For physical photos, use clear bags, envelopes or a box to create the initial 'home'. These are easy solutions to produce in a hurry so you can organise your photos without worrying about storage. Digitally, the organisation comes from categorisation.*

Storage *Printed photos need a home. Designate a space in your home for your photo collection. This could be as simple as assigning a drawer. Or you could purchase photo boxes which have dividers in them so that you can label up the dividers and place your group of photos inside. They are stylish enough to have out on display in the home and will store your photos until you have the time to transfer them to albums or frames.*

KIDS' ARTWORK

In your office (and toy room and kitchen) you will come across your children's works of art. Kids' artwork can be tricky to get to grips with. Young children come home from school, delighted with their cute creations. You put whatever you can on the fridge or walls and the rest is left to one side. The artwork can grow and grow and grow. Parents really struggle with letting artwork go. Whether it's pride in the creativity, guilt that you didn't reward their efforts enough or sadness that they're growing up, it leads to keeping *a lot* of artwork.

If you're going to be strict enough with it, make sure that the memorabilia box you get is at least A4, if not larger. That way you can include artwork in with their other memorabilia. However, if you think you won't be strict with it and you'll be keeping a lot, it will need storage all of its own. There are various

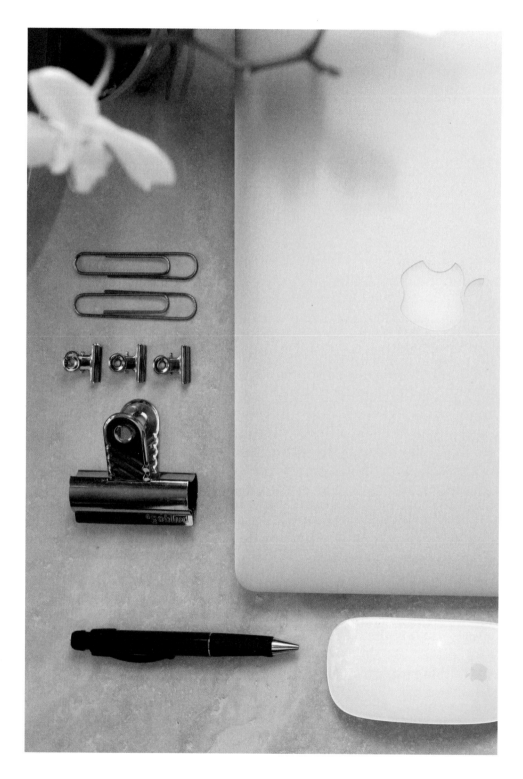

solutions for that. If you're under time pressure, get a large storage box and put all artwork you find in there. You could get one storage box for each child.

If you'd like to develop a nicer system, then why not use a system based on suspension files?

Use a storage box or banker's box with suspension files inside. Or get a large (sturdy) expanding file with suspension files/pockets incorporated inside. Each pocket or file could represent a different year of school. You could use it exclusively for artwork, or you could add in awards, certificates, diplomas, school reports, etc. If you can allocate one system to each child it will be even more organised and provide more space. If you're planning to keep a lot of artwork, you could stick to a large container for that and use the suspension file idea for all other achievements.

With any storage you choose, you need to remember that artwork can be anything from scribbles on some printer paper to an A3 collage to Hallowe'en masks and life-size cardboard Easter bunnies. Your storage needs to accommodate all shapes and sizes.

❹ STORAGE

There is so much office storage out there and if you shop well you can get fun, colourful storage. No more dull green, grey and black storage. If you love stationery, prepare to fall in love with how you can organise it!

Floor space is essential, so choose your large storage carefully. If you already have a filing cabinet and desk in the space, what else can you realistically fit that will improve the function of the room rather than hinder it?

FILING CABINETS

If you choose not to scan your paperwork, and even if you do, you will probably need some sort of filing cabinet. The size needed will differ from office to office. Getting a filling cabinet working well is very important – especially if you're in business. Keeping your paperwork in order will help your productivity, speed up your administration and help with your tax affairs, giving you peace of mind.

Filing cabinets come in a variety of sizes and can be either vertical or horizontal. Vertical filing cabinets take up the least floor space, so if you're stuck for space, go vertical.

DRAWER ORGANISERS

Organisers come in a variety of sizes and you can choose them according to your drawer size. Some organisers stack, which is particularly useful for storage on your desk. They are essential for all your tiny supplies – staples, paperclips, Post-it notes, pens, erasers, pencil sharpeners, highlighters, rubber bands, etc. They are also excellent if you have arts and crafts in a drawer. Small embellishments sit well in drawer dividers.

STORAGE FOR CABLE MANAGEMENT

To hide extension plug sockets and cords, try using a cable box. Cable clips and cable wraps keep wires together. Cable catchers can be stuck to your desk and stop your phone charger and other wires falling down the back of the desk.

If you are on a budget, use clear sandwich bags instead. Place USBs in one, cables for the camera in another, wires from the TV in another and label accordingly.

MAGAZINE FILES AND TACKLE BOXES

Magazine files will, of course, store your magazines, but they are also good for storing notebooks, coloured card, folder dividers, laminator paper, photo paper, printer paper. These items store vertically in a magazine file.

Tackle boxes are excellent if you are keeping arts and crafts on a shelf.

ZIPPED MESH POUCHES

If you don't want or need structured storage, pouches of various sizes are useful. The extra large ones are good for holding artwork; small ones can hold business cards. As they are made of mesh, they are flexible, so you can fit in more than you could in a rigid drawer divider. You also have the choice of storing them lying flat in a drawer or upright on a shelf.

NOTICEBOARDS

Noticeboards are great for reminders or for inspiration. But only if you are actually using them for this. They are highly visual so when there's a lot on them this can become clutter. If you can't find anything on them or aren't feeling very inspired, do you really need them?

STORAGE FOR RECEIPTS

Receipts need to be contained in every office. There are several options:

- CLEAR PLASTIC BAG: One per month, labelled accordingly

- ENVELOPES: One per month, labelled accordingly

- SMALL EXPANDING FILE: a pocket for each month

- PAPER SPIKE

AND MORE

- PENCIL CUPS: Essential on a desk top. But one — you only need one.

- SHALLOW TRAY: For keys, USB sticks, coins, loose paperclips

- PAPER STORAGE: Check out the next chapter for storage solutions to help you tame the paper monster.

Now that you have a grip on the office, what remains is the paperwork. Identify time in your schedule to tackle the paper mountain. If you can stick to the same time each week, all the better. If you can schedule time more often than weekly, better again. It's time to get control of the paper clutter, and time is of the essence!

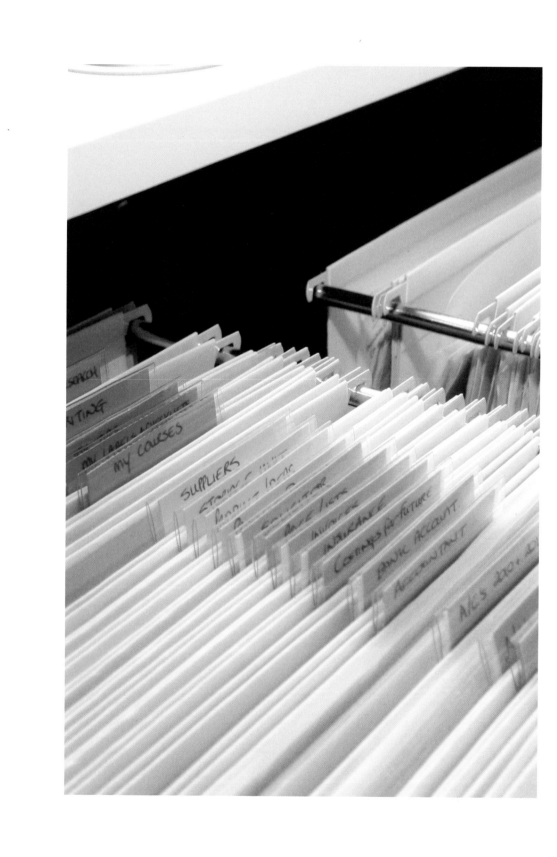

17

PAPER

•

AN ENTIRE BOOK COULD BE
WRITTEN ON ORGANISING PAPER

•

In spite of the rise of the digital age,
with electronic billing, electronic forms,
shopping online, Kindles, iPads and Androids,
paper is still holding its own. This paper has to
go somewhere. And 'somewhere' is on our desks,
in our handbags and cars and on our kitchen
counter tops.

•

Unless dealt with effectively, piles and piles of paper can build up throughout the house, which can be very claustrophobic. Seeing paper build up causes stress, as there is a constant visual reminder that the issue is not being dealt with and each day, when the post arrives, it only gets worse!

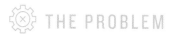 ## THE PROBLEM

Paper clutter is extremely oppressive. The more the paper builds up, the more guilty you feel about not getting it sorted. The more out of control you feel. You feel as if you're surrounded by paper. You're not sure where to start, what to throw out and how to organise the paper you're keeping.

There's every sort of paper here. From receipts to recipes, school notes to bills. It spreads everywhere, gathering on kitchen counter tops, on your bedroom locker, inside kitchen cabinets, in unlabelled folders, in handbags and school bags, in the glove compartment of the car, even in the bread bin or the microwave.

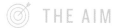 ## THE AIM

Here are some of the goals of an organised paper trail.

- An easy filing system that allows for quick retrieval.

- Understanding exactly what paper you have and why you're keeping it.

- No issues around important paperwork for either yourself or for family members in an emergency.

- A clear system for paper associated with any personal interests and hobbies that allows you to indulge, develop and learn new skills.

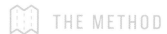 ## THE METHOD

It's important to try to stick with one place for paper. While the ultimate goal is to have one place to store all the paper long term, initially this may not be possible.

In the meantime, as you are organising paper, try to corral it as much as possible. For instance, if you have paper spread on your kitchen counter tops and kitchen island, and some on the table and more down the side of the couch, gather it all up together and choose one area for paper. Simply pile the paper and place it in one spot, perhaps in a corner of the kitchen counter. This is now 'home' to paperwork. Now you just have one pile to deal with. It might be quite a big pile, it may need work, you mightn't know what paper is in the pile, but it's a lot easier to manage and it's better to look at one pile rather than paper scattered over your surfaces and in every nook and cranny.

Do the same in every other room where there is paper. Go up to your bedroom and create one pile of paper there. Go to the utility room and gather any paper in there – probably manuals – and place them all together in one spot. In your office, gather any loose paper, pile it and place it in one spot. If you feel like taking other paper piles from around the home into the office, go for it. The fewer paper nooks around the house, the better.

This is organising without actually organising anything at all. You're simply making it more manageable. When you come to organising and decluttering it properly you will know exactly where to find all the paper. If you find you're missing something during this process, instead of searching everywhere, you now only have a few piles.

By creating these piles you are in effect creating your *backlog*. All this paper will eventually be examined, but for now it's under a little more control and we can move on.

PAPER LIFE CYCLE

When we think about how to organise our paper, we have to think about its *life cycle*: what happens to the paper we accumulate and how we deal with it from the moment it arrives in our home to the moment it goes out again. It comes into our lives in various ways, and a lot of the time you mightn't even notice it coming in. Going back out again involves recycling or shredding.

In between coming in and going out, it hangs around your home and business for you to either use or store. So paper is on a journey and we determine its route and stop-offs along the way. Paper has a tendency to get lost if left to its own devices, which only causes us stress. So put yourself in the driving seat and let paper sit in the back and do what it's told!

RECENT PAPER VS BACKLOG

Everyone thinks that when they start to organise their paper, they need to deal with the backlog. They look around their office, kitchen counter or bedroom floor at all the paper and don't know where to start.

Well, don't start with the backlog. First, you need to deal with the paper that has come in today. And tomorrow, you need to deal with the paper that comes in tomorrow. You need to set up a system and work with the most recent paper. Once that's under control, then you'll move onto the backlog.

Now I understand that your most recent paper could well be mixed up with years of other paper. That credit card bill you need to pay is covered by kids' artwork, pension information, recipes, magazine cut-outs, your club membership. It's all a mess. It's okay. Just focus on the recent paper and it will all unfold (forgive the pun!).

The reason why I suggest starting with the recent paper is because this is the paper you are most likely to need and by extension this paper is more likely to cause stress than older paper. Furthermore, any system you set up for dealing with your most recent paper will be replicated for more long-term paper and for the backlog.

SHORT-TERM VS LONG-TERM STORAGE

There are two systems with paper: short-term filing and long-term filing. Paper that is filed for the short term will eventually make it to long-term filing unless it is thrown out completely. All long-term paper should eventually be thrown out. Let's look at a few examples of this.

FILING PAPER	ACTION
A note comes in from the school with information on holidays and significant school events for the coming school year. No action is needed, but regular reference is required.	L/T SOLUTION
Your health insurance policy comes in the post and is up for renewal. You need to call them and ensure you're happy with the cover. Therefore there is a to-do with this piece of paper and you will need access to it to deal with it.	S/T SOLUTION
The health insurance policy is subsequently dealt with and renewed. There is no further action, but reference may be required over the next year.	L/T SOLUTION
You get a gift voucher/supermarket vouchers in the post. You need access to these.	S/T SOLUTION
Your bank statement comes in the post. There is no action on them but you may need to refer back to them. And you will need to send them to your accountant for year-end returns.	L/T SOLUTION
You get an interiors magazine. You're planning to redecorate and have loads of ideas from various sources. This is not immediate but you'd like to be able to enjoy the design of it and have access to the inspiration.	L/T SOLUTION
The house you live in was a self build. All work is complete, but you need to keep the paper for the work that was done.	L/T SOLUTION
Your baby gets a vaccination and the doctor gives you a vaccination card and information. Aside from health checks, there is no other reason for needing this paper.	L/T SOLUTION
You buy a new iPad. There is a guarantee and instructions inside. Chances are they won't be required, but they need to be kept.	L/T SOLUTION
The pipe between your home and your neighbours' was blocked. You are disputing the cost of getting it fixed. The receipt and other paperwork is needed until it's resolved.	S/T SOLUTION

As you can see, almost every short-term piece of paper is recent and has an action connected with it. Another way of looking at it is as follows:

- Paper that comes in and you've no time to deal with it needs a *short-term* solution.

- Paper that has an action associated with it needs a *short-term* solution.

- Paper relating to action that has started, is in progress but unfinished needs a *short-term* solution.

- Paper that doesn't require action but you need regular access to needs a *long-term* solution.

- Paper that doesn't require action, you don't need regularly but need to keep for future reference needs a *long-term* solution.

The main issue with getting control over paperwork is the actions associated with it: the to-dos. Some paper we just need for reference, but a lot of paper involves a task and we leave it out to remind ourselves of that. Therefore, to organise your paper, you have to organise your time. If you can't shift the to-dos that come with the paper, you won't be able to shift the paper itself.

Systems are needed to conquer this. Which is why we need a short-term paper system and a long-term paper system. If you can get the hang of this, you'll be well on your way to organising paper.

SHORT-TERM SYSTEM

STEP 1. CREATE A SOLUTION

Choose one spot in your home that will from now on be the place to put all new incoming paper. Buy a letter tray, a basket or simply any sort of shallow empty box that you can use to put any *new* paper that comes into your home. This box *must* be shallow. If you use a large or deep box, it'll be weeks or months before it fills up. A shallow box will fill up more quickly, which will force you to file away your paper.

Tomorrow morning, when the post arrives, instead of mindlessly throwing it anywhere, *mindfully* place it in this box or tray.

You have now created your *recent* paperwork.

STEP 2. CREATE A DAILY HABIT

Every day you will be more aware of exactly where you are putting paper. Every day, all types of paper – school circulars, bills, appointment notes, cards, receipts – will be collected in this one spot. This is a new habit and a new system. Now, if anyone is searching for a recent piece of paper, there is only one place it could be.

What makes dealing with paperwork difficult is that often we are not sure what we are looking at or where we left off with each piece of paper. Time is taken up with trying to figure out what we were supposed to do next with the piece of paper in our hands. This is such a waste of time, it can overwhelm us and can lead to poor decisions. As paper comes into your life, you may not have time to deal with it immediately. This happens nine times out of ten. There is always going to be paperwork that you can't get around to putting away. There is always going to be paper that is currently needed for your daily life. And there is always going to be paperwork that you need out in order to get things done. For example:

- You've come in from a morning shopping, and your wallet is full of receipts that you don't have time to file.

- You got the bathroom remodelled but there's a problem with the plumbing. You need to keep your invoices to hand as you make arrangements to get this fixed.

- Your child has a birthday party at the weekend and you bought a card and wrapping paper for the present. The receipt is lying around too.

- There's a new Pilates class starting in the community centre, and you keep meaning to book your place. The leaflet is left out as a reminder.

All this paperwork has a valid reason for being out. But it needs a temporary solution to stop it spreading.

The basket or box for the incoming paper is the solution. But you can make this work better for you.

First, staple together pieces of paper that belong together. This in essence makes it one piece of paper and important information is less likely to get separated and lost.

Second, use a Post-it note to quickly write down what you need to do with it next. Then leave it in the basket.

When you do have time to deal with the paper, you will know exactly what you need to do. No worries and no wondering.

Steps 1 and 2 are the beginning of the short-term system for paperwork organisation. If you follow these steps every day, it will eventually become a habit.

What happens when the basket gets full? What about all the to-dos that come in with the paper? That's when we need Step 3.

CREATE A WEEKLY HABIT

As I've mentioned, organising paper can't be achieved without looking at your time too. In order to continuously clear paper, you have to continuously clear your to-dos. This may be a lot at first, but, trust me, it settles down. The sooner you commit to the time it will take to set up systems and clear the backlog, the quicker it will settle down. It's like losing weight … paper weight.

The weekly system I suggest is:

- ✓ ONCE A WEEK, BRING THE BASKET CONTAINING ALL THE PREVIOUS WEEK'S PAPER TO A DESK OR TABLE. YOU COULD EVEN DO THIS IN FRONT OF THE TV.

- ✓ MAKE SURE YOU HAVE YOUR ORGANISING SUPPLIES TO HAND, A NOTEPAD FOR YOUR TO-DO LIST AND YOUR SCHEDULE – WHETHER IT'S PAPER OR DIGITAL.

- ✓ TAKE THREE POST-IT NOTES AND WRITE 'TO FILE' ON ONE, 'TO DO' ON THE NEXT AND 'TO THROW OUT' ON THE THIRD.

- ✓ WHEN YOU FIND PAPERS YOU DON'T NEED, PUT THE 'TO THROW OUT' POST-IT ON TOP OF THEM.

- ✓ WHEN YOU FIND PAPERS THAT YOU DON'T NEED TO DO ANYTHING WITH BUT NEED TO KEEP, PUT THE 'TO FILE' POST-IT ON TOP OF THEM.

- ✓ WHEN YOU FIND PAPERS THAT YOU NEED AND HAVE TO BE ACTIONED, PUT THE 'TO DO' POST-IT ON TOP OF THEM AND WRITE THE ACTION ON YOUR TO DO LIST.

Once you have gone through each piece of paper, you will have:

1 A TO-DO LIST

2 A BUNDLE OF PAPER FOR THE BASKET (TO DO)

3 A BUNDLE OF PAPER FOR LONG-TERM STORAGE (TO FILE)

4 A BUNDLE OF PAPER FOR THE BIN (TO THROW OUT).

THE TO-DO LIST

The paperwork will form a large part of your daily to-do list. In Part II we created these to-do lists. Now, with this paperwork, more tasks are added on. As we saw, we prioritise the tasks and add them to the schedule.

Taking each of these tasks, look across your week and find a good time to get the tasks done. Look at activities already in your schedule. Then compare your week with the to-dos and see where you can slot them in. When you come to do the task in your schedule, you will have the corresponding piece of paper you need in the basket.

THE BASKET

The paper in the basket is current. It is either for reference or matches a to-do that you will schedule. As the week goes on, more paper will be added here. It will be treated in the exact same way. You will see to-dos getting finished, paperwork moving on to the bin or to filing, and new paperwork coming in. This is the paper life cycle. But the most important thing to note is that *all* paper here is *current*. It's either brand new information or it's in progress.

At this stage you will note that the basket works in conjunction with the to-do list. **Basket + to-do list + Habits = Short-term System**

THE BACKLOG

The paper you're finished with and that needs filing is added to your backlog paperwork. Eventually there will be no backlog and the paper will simply be filed away. But for the moment, at the starting line, there is some backlog and this paper will be added to it. Paper here has now moved on to the long-term system.

THE BIN

Get rid of unnecessary and un-needed paper with gusto!

If you do Step 3 each week and factor it into your time management routine, you will move your to-dos off the list and move paper to long-term filing or to the bin.

The system is repeated, tasks get done and paper reduces week in, week out. Eventually, you will be on top of your to-dos and paper and you will find you can ease the system out to twice a month or monthly.

LONG-TERM SYSTEM

Sorting through the backlog is going to take some time. It is best to have a large, clear floor space or large table (maybe a dining room table) where you can not only spread paper out, but also leave it from one organising session to the next. As paper is decluttered and sorted, the same categories will appear time and time again. If, for instance, you find some bank statements in one pile and you create a 'bank statements' category, it would be easier to leave this out for the duration of your work so that as you move through all the paper, each time you find a bank statement, you can simply add it to the correct category.

You need to be neat and conscientious at this point. It's essential to have a place in your home where you can keep this newly organised and categorised paper together. You've started your temporary system, and you don't want it to come undone while it's in progress.

At your next session, you can pull it all out again, continue to go through your backlog and build on the categories.

The creation of the long-term system uses the same steps that you have seen in earlier chapters on organising the rooms in a home. So let's get stuck in!

❶ CATEGORISE

- Take a bundle of paper.

- Look at the first sheet. What is it? What's the first word that comes to mind? Write that down. Don't over-think it. Don't think you're wrong. Whatever description pops up in your mind when you look at the paper, use that. For example: a credit card bill. What do you think when you look at it? Do you think Credit card? Or Visa? Or Bank? Whatever it is, that's your category. Or a TV licence notice. Do you think TV licence? Or Television? Or Home? Or Utilities? Whatever it is, that's your category.

- When you decide on the word, you have created a category. Fold an A4 piece of paper around the paper you are dealing with and on the front write down the description that you came up with.

- Take up the second piece of paper. What is it? What do you think of when you look at it? Write that down.

- Take a folded piece of paper and wrap it around the paper you are dealing with. Write the description on the front. This is your second category.

- Take the next piece of paper and do the same. The piece of paper may fit into a new category, or it might make sense to add it to a category you've already created.

- Have a designated spot for paper to be recycled/binned/shredded to one side.

- If you have two or more pieces of paper that belong to each other, staple them.

Repeat the process for each piece of paper.

When you first start decluttering, many categories may emerge. However, the further into the piles of paper you go, you will see dominant types of paper repeating. By the end, smaller categories can be assimilated into a larger one that makes sense. To keep track of the categories, writing them down may help. As it will take you several sessions to get through the paper, you may forget how you were categorising a document from one session to the next.

Examples of categories that emerge for paperwork include:

HOME	WORK
Insurance	Finance
Bank	Marketing and PR
Credit card	Recruitment & training
Personal	Sales
Health	Client information
Car	Research
Kids	Forward planning
Photographs	
School work	
Artwork	
Utilities	
Rent/mortgage	
Second property	
Pension	
Research	
Reading	
Inspiration/motivational	
Home extension	
Plans	
Memorabilia	
Loose receipts	

CREATING SUB CATEGORIES

All the above categories are examples of one-tier categorisation. This is the quickest and easiest way to whittle through paper and categorise it in order to file. However, sometimes, you may need to sub-categorise.

For example, you have insurance papers for car, home and health. In a straightforward one-tier system, you'd categorise and file all insurance papers under 'insurance'.

However, if you want to specifically identify car, home and health, then you sub-categorise into a two-tier system. For example:

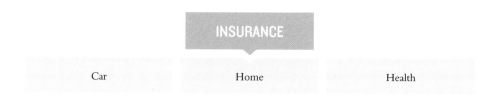

INSURANCE

Car   Home   Health

Similarly, with financial documents, you might put everything under 'bank' and that's a one-tier system. Or you may like to sub-categorise, as I have done below.

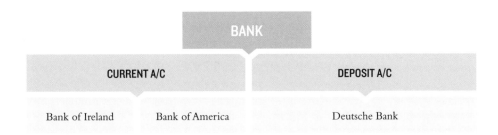

Another example is organising children's paperwork, where you can do something similar. In a one-tier system, you would put everything for Sophie into one file. Or you can organise it further into a tiered system.

SOPHIE		
SCHOOL	HEALTH	IMPORTANT DOCUMENTS
Reports Friends	Tests Receipts	Birth Cert Passport

Creating a tiered system with paper can be tricky, so keep it simple if you are surrounded in paper or stuck for time. If you do attempt it, always start with the overall category i.e. the first tier; then all other tiers drop down from that.

❷ DECLUTTER

We already know that clutter builds up when we don't make a decision on it and paper is no exception.

Some of the reasons why decisions on paperwork are difficult and we procrastinate are because managing paper is boring; you can think of 16 different ways you could file each piece of paper; uncertainty. Being more aware of this should help.

Yes, it's boring – so put a time limit on it. This will help you stay focused. Yes, there may be 16 different ways to file. But what was the first solution that came into your head? Use that. Yes, there's uncertainty. We can put systems in place to help, but there will always be some level of uncertainty.

LIFE CYCLE OF A PIECE OF PAPER

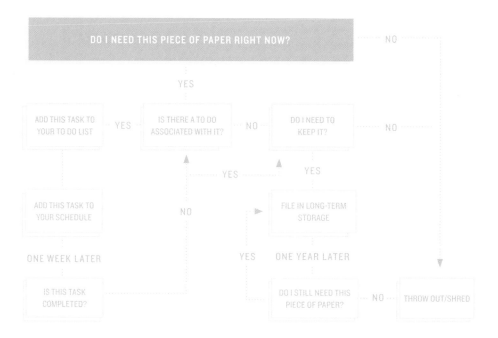

To help with decisions, every time you have to deal with paper and need to make a decision on it, follow this chart. It will help you find a home for every piece of paper that you own, leading you to either the short-term system or the long-term system.

As you move through the backlog, you will find tasks you were supposed to do ages ago. Take a Post-it and write what you need to do next on it. Add the paper to the basket in your short-term system. If it's particularly urgent, look at your schedule for today and see what can you move around to accommodate it. If it's not urgent, deal with it during your weekly time management routine, adding it to a to-do list and scheduling it in next week.

PAPER TO KEEP LONG TERM

If you are a sole trader and need to complete annual tax returns, financial and important documents need to be kept for six years, plus the current year, before they can be destroyed. For others, the rules are more lax. However, there are some documents everyone needs to keep. And if you are unsure, check with your bank, accountant or solicitor. These documents are:

- ✓ ANNUAL TAX RETURNS (FOR BUSINESSES)

- ✓ DEEDS, MORTGAGES, BILLS OF SALE

- ✓ REAL ESTATE CERTIFICATES

- ✓ HOME IMPROVEMENT DOCUMENTS

- ✓ RECEIPTS FOR MAJOR PURCHASES (TO ACT AS WARRANTIES/GUARANTEES)

- ✓ WILLS, LIVING WILLS

- ✓ MEDICAL AND BURIAL INSTRUCTIONS

- ✓ POWER OF ATTORNEY INSTRUCTIONS

- ✓ PENSION INFORMATION/RETIREMENT PLANNING

- ✓ BIRTH, MARRIAGE AND DEATH CERTIFICATES

- ✓ DIVORCE PAPERS

- ✓ PASSPORTS

- ✓ INVESTMENT RECORDS

- ✓ VEHICLE TITLES

- ✓ CURRENT INSURANCE RECORDS – HOME, CAR, HEALTH

- ✓ MEDICAL RECORDS

❸ ORGANISE

Any paper you need to keep will need a long-term filing solution(s). You probably already have some of these solutions. Expanding files, lever arch folders and filing cabinets are the usual solutions for paper. If you do use these solutions but they are now full, it's best to sort them out before you move to your backlog. Yes, leave the backlog until last. There is no point organising that if the paper has nowhere to go. It's what got you here in the first place.

Below are the main filing solutions when you need to keep paper long term. There are positives and negatives to bear in mind. The most important factor to consider is how good you think you're going to be at getting rid of paper. Not so good? You will need a lot of storage.

❹ STORAGE

STATIONERY

Every office needs the following items. These items will help you organise your paper.

- ✓ SCISSORS
- ✓ PAPERCLIPS
- ✓ STAPLER
- ✓ STAPLES
- ✓ STAPLE REMOVER

- ✓ HOLE PUNCH
- ✓ PRITT STICK (OR SIMILAR)
- ✓ SELLOTAPE
- ✓ BLU TACK

- ✓ ELASTIC BANDS
- ✓ PRINTER PAPER
- ✓ BULLDOG CLIPS – LARGE AND SMALL
- ✓ L-SHAPED PLASTIC POCKETS

FILING CABINETS

Filing cabinets are good for large volumes of paper. They are also the quickest solution. If you hate filing, simply popping paper into an organised filing cabinet is the quickest and easiest solution.

Good for: all types of paper – home or business.

If you really want to bring your filing cabinet to life, then here's how and *why* you should colour-code your filing system. A lot of people do go down the colour-coding route when organising paper, for instance green for finance, blue for utility bills, red for files that need attention.

There is one problem with organising this way if you want to maintain the system long term.

Generally, when you buy suspension files, the manufacturers determine for you the number of green/red/yellow, etc, files in a pack. Let's say you decide to allocate your green folders to finance, but the pack you buy only has two green ones and you need four. So you need more green files for your finances. What do you do then? Buy more? That could be annoying to do, time-consuming and expensive.

Or you do have enough of the different-coloured files, but files will break. You go off to buy more of the same colour to keep the coding in sync but they've discontinued the type of file.

So if you're using suspension files, stick to the same file colour and show the category colour on the tab instead. If you identify the paperwork category by the colour on the tab and not the suspension file itself, should you need to change the filing in any way, your files will always be uniform and it's a lot less hassle to change the label.

In my filing cabinet I use white throughout. To show the colour code, I added coloured Post-it notes over the tab to differentiate the categories of paperwork. Suspension files with a green tab are finance sub-categorised into tax, accountant, bank statements. Suspension files with a purple tab are PR sub-categorised into social media, radio interviews, articles I've written, etc. So when I open my filing cabinet, my eye is drawn to the category I need because I remember the colour. I don't have to rifle through any other file or category type.

Finally, some files can get pretty big and can make even the nicest filing cabinet look messy. In this instance, I find putting a bulldog clip over the suspension file helps keep paper in place. It also gives the file a little extra strength. And it looks really nice!

EXPANDING FILE/ACCORDION FILE

If you don't have large volumes of paper, an expanding file is a good choice. They work on the same principle as a filing cabinet, but are much smaller and more compact if you're stuck for space.

Good for: home administration paperwork, kids' paperwork (school notes, reports, health details).

BOX FILES

If you use these, place a table of contents at the front so you can clearly see upon opening what's inside without having to rummage. Make sure to label clearly. If you need more than one box for a certain category of paperwork, make sure to label 'Box 1 of 3', 'Box 2 of 3', etc.

Good for: property portfolio details, pension details, memorabilia (paper), equipment manuals.

LEVER ARCH FOLDERS

Finally, lever arch folders, or folders with pockets, are another choice. They are the most common form of filing, a hangover from our schooldays. Some people like folders as you can clearly see what's inside by flicking through the pages. However, I find them cumbersome. If you want to file paper quickly, these are not for you. The paper can rip, as can the plastic pockets, which in turn affects their ability to keep you organised. They also only hold a limited amount of paper.

If you do use them, label the outside, place a table of contents at the front, and use extra wide dividers with the pockets so you can see the divisions clearly.

Good for: school subjects (one folder per subject), snippets of business/PR information.

MIX AND MATCH

When choosing storage, it is possible to mix and match your solutions. For example, I have a large filing cabinet for my business paperwork, an expanding file for my home paperwork, a box file for pension details, etc. You could do this too. For example, you could home all your family administration paperwork in an expanding file in the kitchen; the kids could use lever arch folders for school work. It depends on your own aesthetic. What is key is that putting things away and retrieving them should be really easy.

IN SPITE OF
THE RISE OF THE
DIGITAL AGE,
KINDLES, IPADS
AND ANDROIDS,
PAPER IS
STILL HOLDING
ITS OWN.

When paper is good to go, schedule time once or twice a year to get rid of your oldest documents. The end of the tax year, the start of the school year, the new year might all be good times to schedule it in.

Remove the oldest items. This frees up space to move the paperwork from the year just gone in to your archive storage. This keeps the paper moving, organised and always up to date! Oldest paper out, newest paper in.

Finally, always keep the life cycle and the habits around a paper routine in mind:

PAPER IN

↓

SHORT TERM SYSTEM (BASKET + TO-DO LIST + HABIT)

↓

LONG TERM SYSTEM (STORAGE SOLUTIONS + HABIT)

↓

PAPER OUT

Paper is not easy, which is why it is so important to stay on top of it regularly. Don't let any insignificant piece of paper enter your life! Be ruthless with paper. No one wants to spend their evenings sorting through paperwork. However, if you have a lot of it, you've two choices. Either burn it all or sort it. I would recommend doing either option quickly. Whichever option you choose, once the backlog is clear, maintaining it through habit is the only way. Recognise how you are using paper. Be more mindful of the type of paper you regularly have in your life and what you do with it. One way or another, everyone still needs to deal with paper. Stop resisting that fact and accept it. Stop fighting the current and go with the tide.

Disorganised paper isn't the absence of a system. It's the absence of a habit. It's not the system that will save you and create perfectly organised paper, it's your motivation, commitment and regular time allocation that are going to get you there. The system is your support. But success is and always will be down to your approach.

Part IV

Yourself

·

'YOU ARE WHAT YOU
REPEATEDLY DO, SUCCESS
THEREFORE IS NOT AN ACT,
BUT A HABIT.'

ARISTOTLE

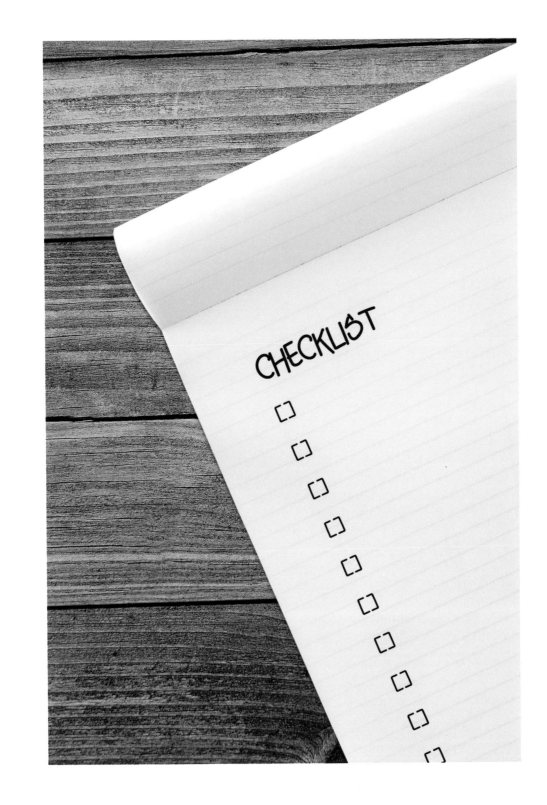

18

ROUTINES &
CHECKLISTS

·

EVERY CLIENT ASKS ME, 'HOW DO I MAINTAIN
THIS?' BEFORE ANY WORK AT ALL IS DONE,
MAINTAINING ORGANISATION IS VERY IMPORTANT
TO THE CLIENT.

·

In this part of the book, we take your goals and
the time you have and create routines so that
you can achieve and maintain a more organised
home, a higher level of fitness, or guilt-free play
time with the kids.

·

What's the point in spending hours or days working at this, only for it to fall to pieces? As we have seen, it's all about our habits. And what makes a good habit stick? A routine. The key to success is in your routines.

You have cleared a large amount of stuff out of your life. You have more space, there is a feeling of relief, you feel you're getting somewhere. You have more energy and feel less overwhelmed.

However, the room will get messy again. The kids will dump their school bags and homework all over the kitchen. You will arrive home from a holiday or business trip and leave the suitcase open in the bedroom. You will accumulate more things. You will buy stuff, acquire stuff, be given gifts. Decluttering will be needed again, but hopefully not for a very long time and it should be much quicker to do next time around.

Ensuring that the mess is quickly tidied up and that decluttering is only needed on rare occasions lies in your ability to create routines and carry them out in a timely fashion.

Routines are key to the success of anything you want in your life. Physical, mental, emotional and financial success all hinge on the routines you create around them. From organisation to fitness, building a business to spending quality time with family, how you habitually spend your time or where you invest your time will determine what level of success you have and what you attract into your life.

Books, podcasts, conventions all provide fantastic information and help your personal development. But then you don't do anything with this information. Even if you do put what you have learned into practice, unless it is routine practice, it won't take hold the way it could. If you habitually take time to exercise, you attract fitness. If you habitually buy stuff but never clear it out, you attract disorganisation. If you only do what you need to do when you feel like it, days slip by and nothing really changes. That's the key – 'when you feel like it'. Too often we just don't bother if we don't feel like doing something. We put it off for another day and slowly fall into a habit of procrastination. Determination, however, is doing what you need to do when you don't feel like doing it. Routines allow us to do what we don't feel like doing, quickly, and allow us to do what we do feel like doing, efficiently!

They say that when you change your habits, you change your life. How do you change habits? Consistency. What offers you consistency? Routines. Routines put the control back in your hands. In a world where you may feel utterly out of control, any level of consistency in your day can do wonders for your mental health. Routines offer discipline and motivation.

Routines are examples of external systems. They reduce the number of distractions in your life. Routines will set you free.

If you are doing the same or similar tasks every day or every week, you need to group them into one time block. This creates a routine. That leads to a habit. We no longer have to think about the tasks at hand. It speeds up the mundane, gets stuff done and gives us back time. It allows you to focus on what you need to focus on without worrying that you are forgetting something or missing out on something.

People sometimes find routines boring, but it's the tasks in a routine that are boring; the routine will speed it all up, if you let it.

WHY BOTHER?

When you are feeling miserable, a routine can help you get the bare minimum done. Often, when you get that much done, it gives you motivation to keep going.

While routines may seem inflexible, as soon as you are without routines in your life, you can feel lost. Great power comes with a routine. When people lose their jobs, they lose not only financial security but also the emotional security that job routine gives. In times of distress and uncertainty, knowing what to do at a certain time each day can help us move forward. We are able to get things done but don't have to think too much in order to do so. The routine around those tasks gives us that freedom.

Motivation is a huge factor in getting anything done. You may decide that today is the day you're going to get up early and go for a run. Or tackle a spare room. Or simply spend an hour cleaning. You may feel incredibly motivated right up to the last minute before you begin. Your head feels clearer than it has in days, you feel more in control and you're raring to go. But when it comes to getting started, your first reaction could be, 'Oh god, why did I agree to this? There are a thousand other things I'd rather do. Can I get out of this?' Your willpower has dropped.

A ROUTINE IS CREATED WHEN YOU GROUP TOGETHER TASKS THAT CAN BE DONE TOGETHER.

If you have a routine in place, you always have the first step to fall back on. *A routine gives you the first step.* Then you do step two, then step three and see how you get on. The routine gives you a physical plan to follow when emotions threaten to take over. This means that you're more likely to stick with the task at hand. The more you stick with it, the more a habit is formed until you no longer have to think about it and it just becomes something you do.

HOW TO CREATE A ROUTINE

A routine is created when you group together tasks that can be done together. You can create this yourself; or you may already do it, just not at the same time each day or week. The key to a routine lies in the time associated with it.

In Part II, assigning 'when' you will do tasks is the crux of getting through your to-do list and reducing your stress. Effectively assigning 'when' to do tasks comes from understanding your schedule.

You may be actively scheduling your week ahead, but you may still be doing some tasks inconsistently. Perhaps one week you add a Pilates class to your schedule, but the next week you're on holidays, and by the time you get back to Pilates and back to adding it into your schedule, a month has passed. While having the class noted in your schedule is great for your time management and a great place to start, doing it consistently is what creates a fitness routine. Adding tasks into the schedule is one level of organisation and does wonders for your time management.

However, if you can ensure that tasks are grouped and repeated at the same time, you bring your organisation up another level through routines. This leads to a habit, which results in saving more time and achieving your goals. In other words, you can add tasks individually into a schedule, but for maximum organisation, you should aim to add routines into your schedule and allow your schedule to accommodate your routines.

Let's say you decide to get the kids to do an hour of chores. The eldest does the vacuuming while the youngest mops the floors. You get them to do it one Saturday morning and the following week you ask them to do it before visiting the grandparents on Sunday afternoon. The following week you forget. What makes this a routine habit is the consistent time associated with the routine. If you are going to group chores together, assign a time too. Kids' chores done every Saturday morning before any weekend fun becomes a weekly routine and develops a cleaning habit. They also appreciate their free time more!

At the moment, you may be putting the dirty laundry on to wash whenever you think of it. When you're at the washing machine, you usually put some clothes in the dryer and fold some garments while you're there. But it's ad hoc, and some days you mightn't get back to the laundry at all. However, if you assign a time, it becomes consistent. Perhaps you'll decide that before leaving the house for the school run, you'll put on the first load of washing for the day. Through a daily routine every morning, you've cleared the backlog by Friday. The daily routine is the system that maintains the organisation of the clothes and the laundry room.

Some routines group tasks that have no similarities except that it's quicker to do one while you do the other. For example, when I empty the dishwasher, I also empty the bins. That's done every second day. That's the time management associated with that routine. Or when I mop the floors, I also change the master bed. Those two tasks have nothing in common except they don't need to be done as often as other cleaning jobs and they take a large amount of time to do. Therefore, I factor them in every two weeks and make sure I have a larger block of time assigned on my schedule for cleaning than I usually need.

Cleaning jobs that need extra muscle or extra time are always bundled together. I'd rather give four hours once a month to get my regular weekly cleaning and my deeper cleaning jobs done than have to do them ad hoc or on the fly throughout the month. I don't mind cleaning, but I don't want to have it hanging over me. I'd rather get jobs done in bulk and move on!

- ✓ **WHAT ARE YOU ALREADY DOING THAT YOU COULD TAG A CLEANING ROUTINE ONTO?**

- ✓ **WHAT ACTIVITIES/TASKS/JOBS DO YOU DO EVERY WEEK?**

- ✓ **WHAT DAY OF THE WEEK OR TIME OF DAY DO YOU DO THEM?**

- ✓ **CAN YOU SEE ANY CONSISTENCY?**

- ✓ **IF NOT, CAN YOU CREATE THAT CONSISTENCY?**

If you have been working on your weekly schedule, it should reveal the answers to these questions for you.

FROM TODAY

Start to incorporate organising and decluttering into your day and week from today.

In Part II, I encouraged you to start writing to-do lists and schedules before your time logs were finished. The same can be done with routines. Routines can be tweaked and improved upon, but no matter how small the change, better to do it sooner imperfectly than later perfectly. Just like making dinner or ringing your mother, a bit of organising has to become part of your day if you want to have a more organised home.

EXAMPLES OF ROUTINES

Below are some examples of the many different routines you can create in your life.

WEEKEND LAUNDRY ROUTINE

- FRIDAY EVENING: wash coloured clothes

- SATURDAY MORNING: wash white clothes, move coloured clothes to dryer (or line)

- SATURDAY LUNCH: wash towels, move white clothes to dryer, add coloured clothes to ironing basket

- SATURDAY AFTERNOON: wash uniforms, move towels to dryer, add white clothes to ironing basket

- SATURDAY EVENING: move uniforms to dryer, add towels to ironing basket

- SUNDAY EVENING: move uniforms to ironing basket, iron contents of basket, put away ironed garments

EVERYDAY ROUTINE

- Make bed

- Wash dishes/load dishwasher

- Clean counters

- Sweep floors

- Tidy living room

- Straighten up couch covers and cushions

- Write tomorrow's to-do list

- Prepare tomorrow's bag

CLEANING AND TIDYING – DAILY ROUTINE

- Clear kitchen island

- 15-minute tidy-up

- Hang up clothes

- Make beds

- Wipe surfaces/counters

- Sweep floors

CLEANING – WEEKLY ROUTINE

- BEDROOM: make bed, open curtains, put away clothes

- HALLWAY: general tidy-up

- LIVING/DINING ROOM: General tidy-up, straighten couch and cushions, clear dining room table

- KITCHEN: wash dishes/load dishwasher, dry dishes/unload dishwasher, tidy and wipe down counter tops, empty bins and disinfect

- BATHROOM: polish mirror, dust surfaces, clean and disinfect sink, bath, taps, toilet, clean floor

CLEANING – YEARLY ROUTINE

- Gutters
- Garden furniture and barbecue
- Windows
- Inside kitchen cupboards
- Window blinds
- Mattresses, duvets and pillows

AFTER WORK/SCHOOL ROUTINE

- Make lunch/supper, tidy up afterwards
- Hang up uniforms
- Clean lunch boxes
- Put uniform out to wash (Friday evening only)
- Start homework

BEFORE DINNER ROUTINE

- Clear homework off kitchen table
- Set table
- Tidy up toys off living room floor

BEFORE BED ROUTINE

- Straighten up family rooms
- Put kids to bed
- Turn off lights, lock up, turn on alarm
- Prepare bag for tomorrow

- Lay out clothes for tomorrow
- Night-time toilette routine

Every January we think about how we're going to improve our lives. We have financial, health, relationship or spiritual goals. Routines are not just for the mundane jobs; they help us to achieve our personal home, work, life goals.

If you work all week and want to spend every second with the kids at the weekend but cleaning the house gets in the way, a routine will help. Clean the house on Saturday morning and forget about it for the rest of the weekend. You can't wish the cleaning jobs away. If you resent having to do it, either hire a cleaner, bring your cleaner in more often or block time out yourself. These solutions involve investing either money or time. Either way, it's an investment you have to make if you want to spend time with the kids.

Whether you want to go on the trip of a lifetime or two weeks in Spain, routines around your finances will get you there. Create routines around reminders to pay bills, checking bank balances, meetings with advisers, updating spreadsheets, organising receipts.

Or take your health. Routines can help here too.

FITNESS ROUTINE

You create a fitness routine when you decide what time in your week you can fit it in and repeat that over several weeks (or for the rest of your life!). For example, you decide you can exercise every Monday, Wednesday and Friday. You've found a Pilates class every Monday evening, and then every Wednesday and Friday you will run before work. There – that's a fitness routine.

However, as we learned in Part II, every task you do involves preparation beforehand and a clear-up afterwards. Bearing that in mind, you can create routines around each form of exercise determined by the time of day you do each. For example:

BEFORE YOUR EVENING PILATES CLASS

- Tidy desk at work
- Write tomorrow's to-do list
- Change into exercise clothes and remove makeup
- Gather supplies – towel, money, bottle of water
- Prepare and eat a snack

BEFORE YOUR MORNING RUN

- Eat a snack
- Get dressed
- Make bed
- Stretch
- Choose podcast/music

AFTER EXERCISE

- Empty gym bag and re-stock for next gym day
- Put dirty clothes into linen bin
- Have shower

You probably do all these things anyway. However, if you write them down and recognise them as a routine, you will assign adequate time to get ready. You don't have to rush, and you won't forget something you need.

Having a routine and knowing exactly what you need to do before exercise makes incorporating fitness into your schedule easier, which in turn helps you stay motivated and encourages you to stick with it.

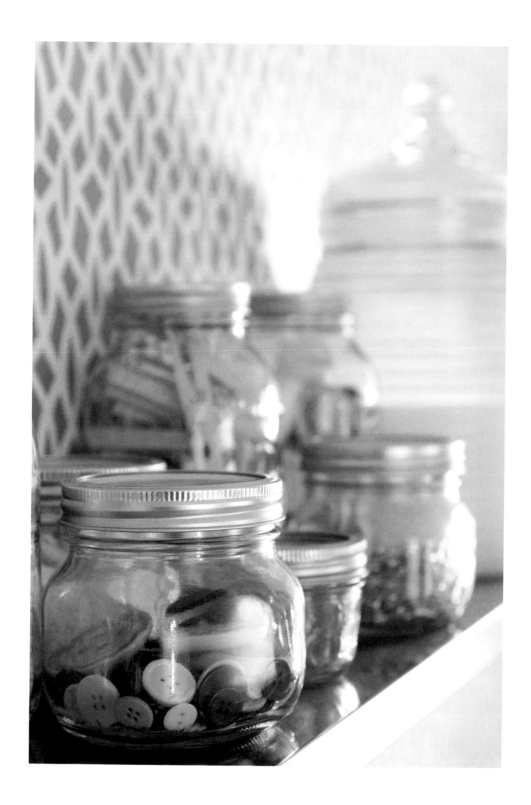

Routines around the clear-up ensure that we get things completed and that organisation is maintained. For example, in the fitness example above, you may feel that as soon as you get home from your Pilates class, that activity is done. In fact, it's not done until you have had your shower and put your gear and towel out to the laundry.

You could flop on the couch as soon as you come in, but then you need to find time for your shower the next morning, which may put you under time pressure. And next week, when your Pilates class comes round, your outfit won't be washed and ready. You have to do these tasks anyway. You have to wash your gym gear eventually. Better to bundle them all in together with the activity they're associated with and get them over and done with.

If you don't acknowledge everything you do around the various activities in your life, it's difficult to stay organised.

MAXIMISING THE MORNING

Mornings, in my opinion, are the most valuable time of day. We never know what is going to happen to us that day, whether things will go as planned or if other more important matters will crop up. Therefore, the morning is the time of day we have the most control over. And this time needs to be used to its maximum.

- What do you regularly not get to?

- What are you dreading and would love to get out of the way?

- Is there something new you'd like to do for yourself?

What about exploring these things first thing in the morning? If you regularly don't get to a household task, would getting to it early in the morning help? Before anyone is awake, before any distractions?

If you are constantly putting off an important work task, one that might actually make a difference to the way you do your job or run your business, getting stuck into it first thing will ease the pressure. For any personal development goals, time in the morning is the secret weapon of some of the world's most successful people.

If you want to take an online course but have no time in the evening, the morning is an option. If you've been thinking about meditating, doing yoga as the sun rises, reading more or writing, there is always an extra 30 minutes if you wake up a little earlier.

Decide what you'd like to do, analyse the preparation and clear-up that would be needed and assign a time every morning or every other morning. Hey presto, you have yourself a new morning ritual. What a lovely way to start your day!

SUNDAY EVENINGS

A good morning routine is backed up by a good evening routine. And none more important than Sunday evening. Transform your week by getting to grips with Sunday night. Make Sunday represent the preparation of a new week. (If you work Tuesday to Saturday this would apply to Monday night.) The evening before your new week is a great time to focus on everything you learned in Part II – List it, Log it, Lay it out.

- Write your Master to-do list.

- Create your Daily to-do lists.

- Fill in your schedule for the next week, including regular activities and upcoming appointments.

- Fill in your schedule with your Top Five priority to-dos.

- Fill in any other to-dos that your schedule will accommodate.

That takes care of your time across the coming week. Then you may add in the following preparation:

- Bags ready (yours and the children's)

- Outfits ready (including any ironing)

- Lunches started

- Transport arranged (money for the bus, organising a taxi, petrol in the car)

- Take a shower

- Set the breakfast table
- Prepare the home:

  → Finishing or starting the laundry cycle

  → Turning on the dishwasher

  → 15-minute clutter clear-up

CHECKLISTS

To take the thinking out of routines completely, write your routine out and you have a checklist. All the steps that make up a routine create a checklist. It's that easy. Every time you need to carry out a routine, follow the checklist. The tasks never change. You follow the steps over and over and over again every time you need to achieve a certain objective.

Checklists are there to avoid forgetting something, avoid repetition of a task and get everything done quickly and efficiently. Checklists keep everyone on track and streamline the process of a project. Any project. From a hospital setting, to health and safety on a building site, from IT security to cleaning your bathroom, checklists get work done.

AVOIDING MISTAKES

Often, certain steps in a project are considered so simple that there is the temptation to skip them or run through them quickly. This can lead to errors. How often have accidents happened as a result of speed or basic mistakes? *Checklists ensure that the basics are done* before you move to the more complex actions.

Mistakes can occur due to miscommunication, late communication, too much information at one time, multiple streams of information and human error. Delays and failures often result from the complexity of a project and the number of people involved. Checklists reduce and often eliminate these issues. The more complex a project, the more essential it is to have a checklist. They keep everyone on the same road to a common goal. If a step is missed, it's noticed. They encourage discipline, but also provide motivation – we all enjoy ticking things off a list. You can also clearly see the project progressing and can see an end in sight as it moves on.

You may feel that checklists are restrictive and don't allow for flexibility; but in fact, a checklist will allow you to tick off the bare minimum and reassure you that you can move on. Personally, I'd feel a lot more creative with that reassurance behind me rather than rebelling against a checklist just because it appears inflexible.

As we have seen, the brain likes to keep things simple. It already has a lot of information it has to process. Checklists reduce that burden on your brain. Checklists reduce pressure all round. It really is as straightforward as 'Here is what needs to be done – follow that and achieve your goal.'

HOW TO CREATE A CHECKLIST

A checklist is created by simply writing down the steps it takes to achieve a certain outcome.

It may be tricky to identify all the steps, but once you do, creating the checklist is very straightforward. You will need a piece of paper and a pen (or a computer and a printer). Simply write a list of numbered steps on the left of the page and add check boxes at the right of the page. If the checklist is for a daily objective and you don't want to print five or seven checklists (one for each day), add five or seven rows of check boxes on the right of the page. Make sure your handwriting is legible, and keep to the same colour ink. Keep checklists together and/or where they are needed most.

FROM TODAY

Don't worry about creating a perfect checklist. Get started – you can fine-tune as you go along. If it's quicker to type it, type it. But it's more important to create a basic checklist and start using it than delay using it because you're perfecting this piece of artwork! Just get it down on paper, start using it and start letting it help you. When you get more time, you can improve it.

CHECKLISTS FOR KIDS

To stay organised during the busy school year, creating systems around the family's routines and habits can really help. Developing a routine and creating a checklist for the kids to follow may help streamline and calm the morning.

A checklist gives ownership to children. They know exactly what's expected of them and what they need to do. It takes the pressure off you – you don't have to nag and answer questions you've probably answered hundreds of times before. Checklists help develop a child's organisational skills. They offer routine to a child, especially one prone to anxiety. Children can also find them fun to use, especially if a reward on Friday is tagged onto them!

Here's a sample morning routine for a young child.

JOHN'S MORNING ROUTINE	
Make bed	☐
Open curtains	☐
Wash face	☐
Get dressed	☐
Come down for breakfast	☐
Eat breakfast	☐
Put lunch in bag	☐
Brush teeth	☐
Go to the toilet	☐
Put on coat	☐

Any routine mentioned above can be formalised with a checklist. Other checklists you might like to consider are checklists for:

- ✓ TRAVEL

- ✓ PACKING

- ✓ DINNER PARTY

- ✓ WRITING A BLOG POST

- ✓ FILMING A YOUTUBE VIDEO

- ✓ CAMPING

- ✓ GARDENING BY SEASON

- ✓ CHRISTMAS

- ✓ HOME SAFETY

- ✓ MOVING HOUSE

Routines and checklists bring your organisation full circle. *Organisation starts and ends with you.* It starts with an understanding of where you are now, where you want to get to and why. It continues with carving out time to physically do the work. And ends with making the time you carved out into a regular, routine occurrence.

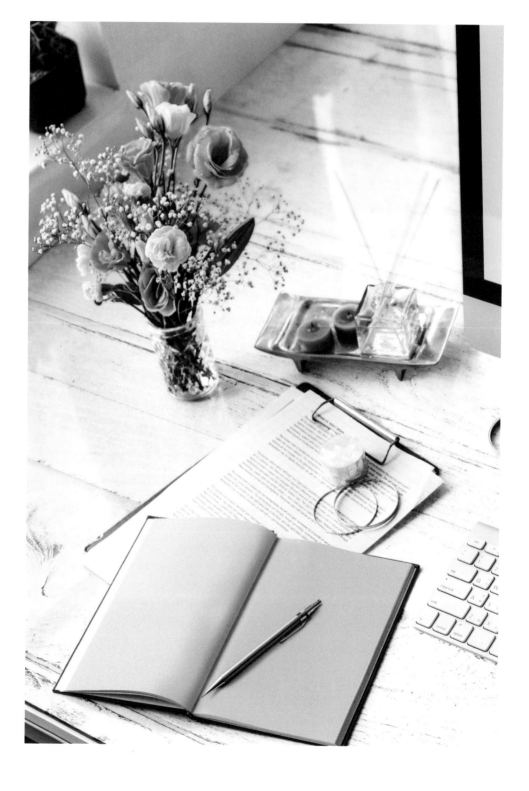

CONCLUSION

·

'DO THE BEST YOU CAN
UNTIL YOU KNOW BETTER. THEN
WHEN YOU KNOW BETTER,
DO BETTER.'

MAYA ANGELOU

·

While writing this book, I often took myself out of my apartment and wrote in nearby cafes and hotels. In the early days of the book, one particular morning, two women were sitting nearby having coffee. Their conversation fell on my ears and while I couldn't make out everything they were saying, I knew they were talking about tidying their homes and the anxiety the mess was causing. Across the noise of the cafe, I caught glimpses into their stress: 'The amount of times I bring home the laptop but … There's always ironing, unless you spend four hours on a Sunday, you'll never get through it … It's not nice, it's not relaxing'. They then mentioned decluttering and tidying the home, and one admitted, 'I'm doing it for my own sanity'.

Throughout this book, I have worked on getting you more space in your home. However, it's the feeling of space inside your head that organisation can bring that will be more important.

When you start to clear space in your home or schedule, you clear space to think. I've had clients start art classes, gardening and yoga, not only because they have more time, but because their brain has had the space to consider it and make it a reality. This in turn brings health, social and personal benefits. Decluttering your life forces you to check in with yourself. Neurosurgeon Dr Henry Marsh in his memoir *Admissions* comments that 'It often seems to me that happiness and possessions are like vitamins and health. Severe lack of vitamins make us ill, but extra vitamins do not make us healthier' (Marsh, 2017, p. 177). Too much stuff has an effect on what we can see around us, and on what we can't see inside us.

We have all held on to things, or people, for longer than we should. It can be upsetting to let go. When you decide to get rid of your possessions, stop focusing on the things that are leaving you. Look instead at what's staying, and focus on the good that's around you. Too much stuff controls us, and even though it's now in a bin bag, you're still focusing on it – worrying if you made the right decision or if you'll regret it.

Why not turn your head to the left or right and look at all the lovely things you're keeping instead? Unless this book has made you Organiser of the Year, I doubt the room is empty. So focus on what's staying; enjoy these things, be grateful.

Don't confuse 'want' with 'need'. We want a lot but we need very little. Our health, physically and mentally, is the number one aspect of our lives that we must appreciate and do anything we can to take care of. There is a greater chance of contentment from owning less than accumulating more.

Decluttering and organisation are a process. If you want long-term results, then learn to enjoy the process more than the outcome. If you declutter your bedroom and then beat yourself up over still having the kitchen, toy room and attic to do, it will be of no help to you whatsoever. With clutter, I am a big believer that time is of the essence. If you decide to do this, then do it. Carve out time in quick succession, stop clutter in its tracks and make some changes. However, you must also remember, as the days or weeks go by, that you are in exactly the place you are supposed to be. Don't look at the next room. Be fully aware, and fully present. Do not resist the struggle; respond to it. It's all in the attitude with which you approach it.

This work can actually be enjoyable. Decluttering is tough sometimes, particularly if you have a lot, or if you're tired. But organising and storage are creating and designing your home, your space, your goals. Not to mention that the results can be beautiful. Have the intention that everything is going to work out well.

Sometimes we can't control what happens to us, but we can always control how we respond. With change, be mindful as you create your new reality, and edit wisely. Respond to periods of stress and allow yourself periods of recovery. Celebrate the ups and keep going through the downs. Enjoy what you accumulate, but recognise when it's time to let go.

And all the while, *breathe in and breathe out.*

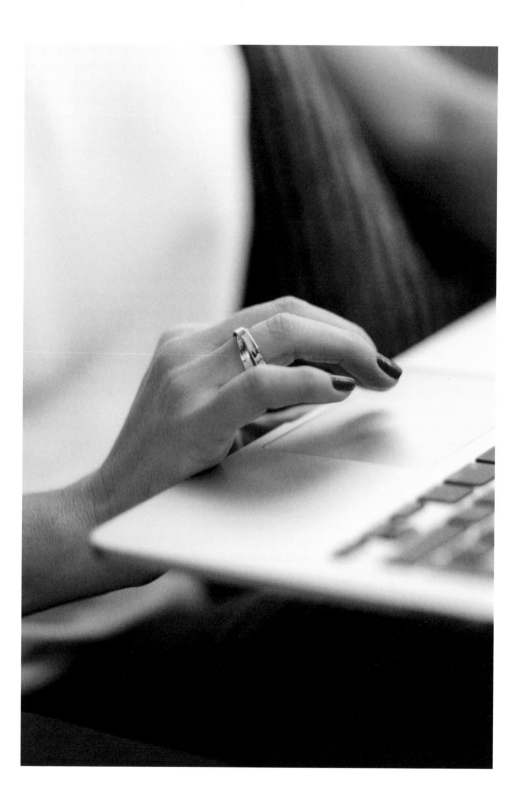

ACKNOWLEDGEMENTS

As I come to the end of writing this book, ironically, I don't want to let it go. Go it must, but not without thanking some people first. I am surrounded by love, help and support and I am delighted to get to acknowledge you all at this point.

Firstly, my thanks to my family. To my mother, Eithne, the kindest person in the world. She always told me to write. To the point of it being annoying. Until one day I listened, and started a blog. She is a wonderful creative writer herself and has helped so many people find their inner author. I can never thank her enough for everything she does and has done for me. Thanks to my Dad, Dermot. He is so generous and has a lovely way of showing how proud he is of me which gives me such encouragement. Thanks to my sister Orla, my cheerleader, who seems to have a never ending stream of creativity coming from her bones! And thanks to my brother David, the funniest person I know and my longest friend. Thank you all for your input into the book, your business ideas, advice, help and love. I love you all very much.

To my extended family. To my wonderful Aunty Niamh and Uncle Noel. To my Aunty Doris, thank you for the help with the business, my Uncle Daire and my grandmother Nora. Thank you.

Thanks to everyone at Gill. It was my dream publisher, and I am so grateful to get the opportunity to work with you and write this book.

Thanks to Sarah Liddy, Commissioning Editor, who recognised just how cool organising is! Thank you for seeing the potential in my script. Thank you for listening to every piece of input I had and welcoming it. I always felt part of the creation of this book beyond the writing, so thank you.

To my editor Sheila Armstrong. Thank you for your all your help. You made it very easy to understand each step of the process and always in such a friendly way. I felt my book was in really safe hands.

Thanks to Esther Ní Dhonnacha, Jane Rogers and Graham Thew. Thanks to Teresa Daly, Ellen Monnelly and Grainne O'Reilly for your ideas and being as enthusiastic about organising as I am!

Thanks to Dr Michael Keane for your time and contribution to the book. Special thanks also to Leslie St Lawrence for the introduction.

Thanks to Ray O'Neill for listening and acknowledging everything. It was needed and has meant a lot.

To the girls, Aine, Catriona, Fiona, Jen, Orna, Roisin, and Siobhan. Friends that have been there for years, always cheering me on and giving advice. You are so important to me. To Joann Bradish, thank you for your kindness, generosity and always being there for me.

My thanks to Hannah Hillyer and Dyann Malcolm. Two gorgeous women who have worked with me to build the business. Their belief in what I do with Organised Chaos has encouraged me to keep going when times were really tough. Thank you for all your help, understanding and support.

Last but by no means least, my thanks to all my clients. You have opened your door feeling nervous, embarrassed and overwhelmed to a person you didn't know, selling something new. I have met such lovely people and heard about such challenges. You trusted me with your stories and your most personal possessions and helped me build a business. I have learnt so much from you. I have learnt gratefulness and resilience through you and the work we have done together. For that, and so much more, I am so very thankful.

REFERENCES

Actualise: Psychological Services and Neurofeedback Training, Dublin City University, www.actualise.ie

Brown, Brené (2012) *Daring Greatly* (Gotham Books, Penguin Group)

Covey, Stephen R. (2004) *The 7 Habits of Highly Effective People* (Simon & Schuster UK)

Duhigg, Charles (2013) *The Power of Habit* (Random House)

Duhigg, Charles (2016) *Smarter, Faster, Better* (Penguin, Random House)

Gilbert, Elizabeth (2015) *Big Magic* (Bloomsbury)

Marsh, Henry (2017) *Admissions* (Weidenfeld & Nicolson)

Levitin, Daniel (2015) *The Organized Mind: Thinking Straight in the Age of Information Overload* (Dutton)

Robbins, Anthony (1992) *Awaken the Giant Within: How to Take Immediate Control of Your Mental, Emotional, Physical and Financial Destiny* (Free Press).

Tindell, Kip, with Paul Keegan and Casey Shilling (2014) *Uncontainable* (Grand Central Publishing)

Vanderkam, Laura (2016) 'How to gain control of your free time' (TED Talk),

http://www.ted.com/talks/laura_vanderkam_how_to_gain_control_of_your_free_time